# Making Sense of Women's Health

## A NATUROPATHIC SOLUTION

D0168097

ActNatural Corporation
5948 3rd Line RR#1
Hillsburgh, ON
N0B 1Z0

ISBN: 978-0-9867247-2-5

Book and Cover Design: Jasper van Meurs
Copy Editing: Susan F. Watts, RN, BScN

Disclaimer:
While all care is taken with the accuracy of the facts and procedures in this book, the author
accepts neither liability nor responsibility to any person with respect to loss, injury or
damage caused, or alleged to be caused directly or indirectly, by the information contained
in this book.

The purpose of this book is to educate and inform. For medical advice you should seek the
individual, personal advice and services of a medical professional.

Printed in Canada by Friesens Corp.

*This book is dedicated to all the amazing women in my life – especially my Mom, whose ongoing support, love and guidance have been my foundation in life. You have helped shape me into who I am today.*

# CONTENTS

# FOREWORD

You don't have to fall victim to your hormonal shifts, as Dr. Marita Schauch explains. Despite all the complexity and the myriad things that can go awry, you can take charge of your health and do it all naturally. From PMS to infertility, fibroids, and menopause, and everything in between, this book explains in plain language what to look for, how to treat it, how to talk to your health care professional about it, and best of all, how to prevent it all from happening in the first place. As we women become more empowered in all spheres of our lives, we also need to understand our bodies, and take charge of our health naturally. On occasion she or I will prescribe medications. However, rather than turning immediately to these powerful, side-effect-laden drugs that only "handle" symptoms, Dr Schauch helps you find the root cause of the problem. With diet, lifestyle, and targeted supplements (herbs, vitamins, minerals) you can then attain a state of balance and harmony.

Hyla Cass M.D., integrative medicine expert, author of *8 Weeks to Vibrant Health: A Take Charge Book for Women to Correct Imbalances, Reclaim Energy, and Restore Well-Being* (www.cassmd.com).

There is an expression in traditional Chinese medicine that says, "to treat one woman is equal to treating five men". This ancient saying highlights the additional intricacies involved in healing women. With our ever-fluctuating hormones, heightened emotional awareness and paradoxically greater tolerance to physical pain, it's no wonder that bringing balance to a woman's wellness seems a daunting task. In short, we women are complex.

But Dr. Marita Schauch shows us that complex doesn't have to mean complicated. If you are sick and tired of being sick and tired, or your intuition is telling you that you should be able to do something to help yourself feel better and you don't know where to start, this book is a good place. By providing a basic understanding of hormones and their actions as well as an insight into principles of naturopathic medicine, Dr. Schauch guides us through a myriad of common women's health concerns and effective natural remedies with straightforward advice.

Kate Rhéaume-Bleue, ND, Canadian health expert and author of *Vitamin K2 and the Calcium Paradox: How a Little Known Vitamin Could Save Your Life* (Wiley & Sons, 2012)

# ACKNOWLEDGEMENTS

I would like to thank Deane Parkes and *Preferred Nutrition* for giving me an amazing opportunity to educate women of all ages. Writing this book has been such an incredible experience.

My family, who continues to shower me with immense support, love and encouragement. My brother Mike, whose keen business sense has taught me that anything is possible with passion, dedication and optimism.

My best friend and loving husband, Markus. Thank you for all your support and patience while I was writing this book. I love you more every day.

I am honoured to be an alumna of the *Canadian College of Naturopathic Medicine* and thank all my naturopathic colleagues for their amazing commitment to educate and promote health and wellness. We are truly blessed to be doing what we do.

Finally, I would like to thank all the women who I have treated in practice - you have challenged me to be a better teacher and doctor. Because of you I am a better person.

# INTRODUCTION

My decision to pursue a career in Naturopathic Medicine was a simple one. I see rapid changes coming to medicine. More and more patients are adopting preventative and proactive approaches to treating their various health concerns. Ten years ago, educating my patients about the principles of Naturopathic Medicine was a part of my regular routine. But in the last few years, I have really seen a shift in the awareness and desire of the general public to look beyond superficial symptoms in order to investigate and treat the cause of disease. Naturopathic Doctors, I believe, are integrating into many health care teams and are offering a complementary approach alongside medical doctors, chiropractors, nutritionists, physiotherapists etc.

I love what I do and I am constantly guided by the six Fundamental Healing Principles of Naturopathic Medicine:

- **First, to do no harm**, by using methods and medicines that minimize the risk of harmful side effects.
- **To treat the causes of disease**, by identifying and removing the underlying causes of illness, rather than suppressing symptoms.
- **To teach the principles of healthy living and preventative medicine**, by sharing knowledge with patients and encouraging individual responsibility for health.
- **To heal the whole person through individualized treatment**, by understanding the unique physical, mental, emotional, genetic, environmental and social factors that contribute to illness, and customizing treatment protocols to the patient.
- **To emphasize prevention**, by partnering with the patient to assess risk factors and recommend appropriate naturopathic interventions to maintain health and prevent illness.
- **To support the healing power of the body**, by recognizing and removing obstacles to the body's inherent self-healing process.

I have always had a passion for educating, researching and treating women's health conditions. In the past few years I have seen an overwhelming increase in hormone-mediated problems especially when it comes to estrogen dominance. The environment is becoming increasingly more toxic and many of these chemicals are very disruptive and harmful to our normal biochemical pathways – especially our hormonal pathways and hormone metabolism. As you will read in this book, environmental chemicals such as Bisphenol-A (BPA), a synthetic estrogen that has been the focus of a growing number of research studies and legislative actions, is detrimental to a woman's body and hormone balance. An estimated 6 billion pounds of BPA are produced globally each year, generating about 6 billion dollars in sales. Just last year, researchers from the Harvard School of Public Health and the Centers for Disease Control and Prevention measured BPA levels in the urine of 244 mothers at various times during pregnancy and in their children at various times after birth. Mothers with higher BPA levels in their urine during pregnancy tended to have 3-year-old girls who were anxious and depressed with poor emotional control and inhibition. A detailed description of the most common environmental toxins can be found in the first chapter on hormones as well as the chapter on breast cancer. In my practice, I have also seen an overwhelming number of cases of infertility and menstrual irregularities. I can't help but wonder if this may be due to increasing environmental insults on the body.

Chronic stress and adrenal function is another passion of mine. Last year, I co-authored *The Adrenal Stress Connection,* a simple booklet on how chronic stress impacts health and the many systems of the body. I chose adrenal fatigue for one of the first chapters in my new book since I believe the adrenal glands play a critical role in hormonal health as well as dictate future disease development. This chapter is a must-read.

*Making Sense of Women's Health* is organized by each woman's health condition. Some women might read it all the way through. Others may find that specific chapter that pertains to their individualized symptoms and health concerns.

As a Naturopathic Doctor, I believe that education is key. You will see each chapter outlined with a description of symptoms and diagnoses of the condition followed by a complementary approach to treatment including dietary and lifestyle tips as well as key supplements for healing.

I have also included a section on conventional medicine as I believe it's important to see both the conventional and alternative approaches to treatment.

I hope that you will find the tools in this book to help you with a lifetime of well-being and good health. Change can be overwhelming at first but start by incorporating one change at a time. You might try to eat more veggies in a day, walk 30 minutes a few times per week or maybe think twice before indulging in dessert after dinner and lunch! By slowly adopting some of the health principles outlined in this book, you can create and nourish a healthier and more vibrant body, mind and spirit.

—————————— CHAPTER 1 ——————————

# HORMONES

## A Delicate Balance

Hormones are powerful chemical messengers that control our mood, energy and stress levels, metabolism, sleep, reproductive function and many other fundamental bodily functions. They function by travelling in the bloodstream and attaching to their specific receptors thus helping to control and regulate the activity of certain cells or organs. To keep all hormones in balance is a challenging task, as hormones are dependent on one another, constantly adapting to accommodate external and internal changes of the body.

## The Endocrine System

The endocrine system is a collection of glands and organs that produce and regulate hormones that help keep the body healthy and balanced. It is derived from the Greek words "endo" meaning inside, and "crinis" meaning secrete. The endocrine system is an information signaling system in which its hormones may be quick or slow to react, with these reactions lasting for minutes, hours or weeks at a time. Below is a summary of some of the major endocrine glands and organs with their hormones and their general functions for keeping a woman's body in equilibrium.

## Hypothalamus

The hypothalamus is located in the middle of the base of the brain. It is responsible for the communication between the nervous system and the endocrine system through the pituitary gland. The hypothalamus controls body temperature, hunger, thirst, fatigue, moods, sleep and circadian cycles.

*Hormones:* TRH, PIH, PRH, GHRH, Somatostatin, GnRH, CRH

## Pineal Gland

The pineal gland is a pea-sized structure buried deep in the brain. Melatonin influences sexual development and sleep-wake cycles.

*Hormone:* Melatonin

## Pituitary Gland

The pituitary gland, often called "The Master Gland", is a protrusion off the bottom of the hypothalamus at the base of the brain. The pituitary gland consists of two components: the anterior pituitary and the posterior pituitary. This gland secretes hormones that regulate homeostasis in the body by working closely with the hypothalamus.

*Anterior pituitary hormones:* Human Growth Hormone (HGH), Thyroid-stimulating hormone (TSH), Adrenocorticotropic hormone (ACTH), Prolactin, Luteinizing hormone (LH), Follicle-stimulating hormone (FSH)

*Posterior pituitary hormones:* Oxytocin and Vasopressin (ADH)

## Thyroid Gland

The thyroid gland is a butterfly-shaped gland that lies across the trachea at the base of the throat, just below the larynx (voice box).

It is one of the larger endocrine glands and controls metabolic rate; meaning how quickly the body uses energy, makes protein, and controls how sensitive the body is to other hormones. It also produces calcitonin, a hormone that plays a role in calcium balance.

*Hormones:* Triiodothyronine (T3), Thyroxine (T4) and Calcitonin

## Parathyroid Glands

The parathyroid glands are four small glands in the neck, located on the rear surface of the thyroid gland. They control the amount of calcium in the blood and within the bones.

*Hormone:* Parathyroid hormone (PTH)

## Thymus

The thymus gland is a specialized organ of the immune system that is located above the heart and behind the upper sternum. It is responsible for the regulation and the development of white blood cells (especially the T cells) in the immune system. The thymus gland shrinks as a person ages.

*Hormones:* Thymosin, Thymopoietin

## Liver

The liver is a vital organ that lies just under the diaphragm, on the right side of the body. It has a wide range of functions, some of which include detoxification, growth, protein synthesis, glucose and fat metabolism, hormone synthesis, lipid digestion and storage.

*Hormones:* Insulin-like growth factor (IGF-1), Angiotensinogen

## Pancreas

The pancreas is located under the left rib cage lying deep to the back. It controls blood sugar levels, breaks down protein, carbohydrates, and fats using its digestive enzymes.

*Hormones:* Insulin, Glucagon, Somatostatin

## Adrenal Glands

The adrenal glands are two walnut-shaped glands that sit on top of the kidneys and are the body's main stress responders. They release hormones in response to stress to help our body adapt. They also help control salt and water balance, regulate sleep and mood, support the immune system increasing resistance to bacteria/viruses, increase libido and maintain normal sex hormone levels, and control inflammation, preventing chronic disease. There are two parts of the adrenal glands: an inner portion (the medulla) and outer portion (the cortex).

*Adrenal cortex hormones:* Aldosterone, Cortisol, Androgens

*Adrenal medulla hormones:* Epinephrine, Norepinephrine also known as Adrenaline and Noradrenaline

## Ovaries

The ovaries are located in the lower abdomen on either side of the groin and control sexual development in women, maturation and release of eggs and fertility.

*Hormones:* Estrogen, Progesterone

## The Normal Menstrual Cycle

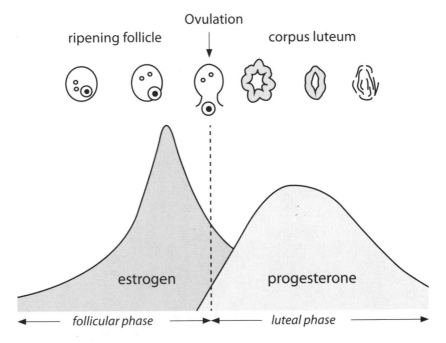

A women's menstrual cycle usually lasts about a month (25 to 35 days), the average being 28 days. It consists of a series of complex hormonal changes and commonly is divided into three phases: Follicular, Ovulation and Luteal. The cycle is under the primary control of:

- Gonadotropin releasing hormone (GnRH) from the hypothalamus
- FSH and LH from the anterior pituitary
- Estrogen and progesterone from the ovary.

## Follicular Phase

During the follicular phase, the dominant hormone is estrogen. The first day of menstruation is Day 1 of a cycle. On average, menstruation lasts from one to five days whereby there is shedding of the uterine lining (bleeding). Estrogen levels begin to increase gradually, thickening the lining of the uterus for the next number of days. Follicle-stimulating hormone (FSH) is released by the pituitary gland leading to the development of a mature egg in the ovarian follicle. When estrogen levels become high, FSH is suppressed leading to the secretion of luteinizing hormone (LH) by the pituitary gland.

Immediately before ovulation, the persistently high levels of estrogen, aided by rising levels of progesterone, enhance pituitary responsiveness to GnRH (from the hypothalamus) increasing LH. This increase is known as the "LH surge" and is an essential part of ovulation. High levels of estrogen in the late follicular phase prepare the uterus for a possible pregnancy. The endometrium (uterine lining) thickens and just before ovulation, the cervical glands produce copious amounts of thin, stringy mucous to facilitate sperm entry. The stage is set for ovulation.

## Ovulation

About 16-24 hours after LH peaks, ovulation occurs. The egg is released from the mature follicle, swept into the Fallopian tube and carried away to be fertilized or die. Estrogen synthesis diminishes.

## Luteal Phase

After the egg is released from the ovary, the ruptured follicle develops into the corpus luteum. The corpus luteum produces steadily increasing amounts of progesterone and estrogen, with progesterone being the dominant hormone of the luteal phase. Estrogen levels increase but never reach the peak seen before ovulation.

Under the influence of progesterone, the endometrium continues its preparation for pregnancy. Progesterone also causes cervical mucus to thicken. Thicker mucus creates a plug that blocks the cervical opening, preventing bacteria as well as sperm from entering the uterus at this time. The corpus luteum has a life span of approximately 12 days. If pregnancy does not occur, the corpus luteum spontaneously degenerates. Without the corpus luteum and the presence of progesterone, blood vessels in the surface layer of the endometrium contract. Lacking oxygen and nutrients, the surface cells die and the lining sloughs off. This begins menstruation.

## Hormone Imbalance

In good health, female hormones work together in a delicate balance. Unfortunately, subtle or obvious hormonal imbalances can cause a multitude of women's health conditions. These imbalances can be triggered by a variety of factors:

- STRESS!
- Poor diet - overabundance of hydrogenated fats, refined sugars and carbohydrates, red meat, dairy, alcohol, and/or caffeine
- Possible food allergies/intolerances
- Vitamin and/or mineral deficiencies
- Congested or sluggish liver impairing proper liver function
- Poor intestinal flora, overgrowth of "bad" bacteria (candida) and not enough "good" (lactobacillus acidophilus and bifidobacterium)
- Smoking
- Exposure to environmental toxins including PCBs, BPA, dioxin, pesticides, phthalates, PVC and parabens
- Birth control pills, hormone replacement therapy, pharmaceuticals
- Heavy metals
- No exercise
- Shift work and insomnia
- Poor body composition (obesity or being underweight)
- Diabetes, insulin resistance.

A list of common hormones, their actions and how their balance can affect a woman's health and well-being are listed below.

## Estrogen

Estrogen is present in both men and women, but in significantly greater quantities in women.

Estrogen is produced in the ovaries (and in the testes in men) and in smaller amounts in the adrenal gland. There are three major naturally occurring estrogens in women: estrone (E1), estradiol (E2) and estriol (E3). They are categorized as "strong" estrogens (estrone and estradiol) or "weak" (estriol). They perform many functions, but chiefly estrogens affect the reproductive system and are responsible for the female characteristics - breasts, menstruation, and pregnancy. The ovaries begin producing estrogen during puberty; and as outlined above in the menstrual cycle, FSH signals the production of estrogen from Day 1 up to the day of ovulation to prepare a woman's body for a possible pregnancy.

### Estrone (E1)

Estrone is the second strongest estrogen and is produced in the ovaries, fat cells and adrenal glands. During menopause, the ovaries shut down and the adrenal glands take over the steroid hormone production. The adrenal glands will produce testosterone and androstenedione in higher amounts, which can be converted into estradiol and estrone in fat cells through the action of the enzyme, aromatase. Estrone is the primary estrogen in postmenopausal women.

### Estradiol (E2)

During the reproductive years, the primary estrogen is estradiol - the strongest of the three estrogens. It is produced mainly by the ovaries, with smaller amounts by the adrenal glands. Higher levels of both estrone and estradiol have been strongly linked with an increased risk of breast, uterine, and ovarian cancers.

*Estriol (E3)*
Estriol is produced in significant amounts during pregnancy as it is made by the placenta. It is a short-acting weak estrogen and can be synthesized from a breakdown product of estradiol and estrone in the liver. Estriol exerts protective effects when it binds to receptors and prevents stronger estrogens such as estradiol, estrone or xenoestrogens (environmental estrogens) from binding and creating unwanted symptoms of estrogen dominance.

## Estrogen Dominance
A variety of women's health conditions (fibrocystic breasts and breast cancer, uterine fibroids, ovarian cysts, PMS, endometriosis, polycystic ovarian syndrome, and hypothyroidism) are often caused by an imbalance of estrogen and progesterone in which estrogen is in excess. This is referred to as "estrogen dominance". Xenoestrogens, excess estradiol and estrone, the birth control pill and hormone replacement therapy all contribute to estrogen dominance in women.

## Estrogen Metabolites C2, C4 and C16
The metabolism of estrogen within the body involves a series of complex reactions that takes place primarily in the liver. Estrogen is broken down through detoxification pathways - Phase I and Phase II - and then is excreted in the urine and stool. Glucuronidation is one of the key Phase II liver detoxification pathways for estrogens and other toxins. It involves estrogen bound to glucuronic acid in the liver. This complex then moves into the intestines and is excreted through the stool. When estrogens are broken down in the liver, several estrogen metabolites are formed. The metabolites are broken down into "good" and "bad" estrogens. C2 estrogens are harmless while C4 and C16 are carcinogenic. The C4 and C16 estrogen pathways are activated by numerous xenoestrogens (which are listed below) as well as poor lifestyle and dietary choices.

## Xenoestrogens and other Hormone Disrupters
Xenoestrogens are man-made environmental chemicals that mimic the

effects of natural estrogens in the body ("xeno" meaning foreign). They are implicated in a number of women's health conditions and can contribute to estrogen dominance. Many of these chemicals not only disrupt female hormones but also affect fertility in both men and women. They are known to increase the risk of cancer and have been implicated in developmental problems in children. You might be surprised to see that many of them are found in our day-to-day activities. Some common xenoestrogens are listed below.

### *Bisphenol-A*

Bisphenol-A (BPA) is a synthetic estrogen used to harden polycarbonate plastics and epoxy resin. There is an estimated six billion pounds of BPA produced world-wide every year. Thousands of products are manufactured using BPA, including safety equipment, eyeglasses, computer and cell phone casings, water and beverage bottles and epoxy paint and coatings. BPA-based plastics can break down, particularly when heated or washed with a strong detergent.

### Tips to Avoid BPA

- Avoid foods such as canned beans, tomatoes, soups and pasta. The cans are often lined with BPA which can leach into the food.
- Use glass water bottles and food containers instead of plastic. Avoid polycarbonate - a plastic that is often marked with the recycling code #7. Plastics with the recycling labels #1, #2 and #4 on the bottom may be better choices because they do not contain BPA.
- Avoid putting any plastic containers into the microwave.

### *Phthalates*

Phthalates ("plasticizers") are a group of industrial chemicals used to make plastics like polyvinyl chloride (PVC) more flexible or resilient. Phthalates are found in toys, food packaging, hoses, raincoats, shower curtains, vinyl flooring, wall coverings, lubricants, adhesives, detergents, nail polish, hair spray and shampoo.

## Tips to Avoid Phthalates

- Read labels and watch for DEHP, DINP, DIDP, DBP, DnOP, DnHP which are all derivatives of phthalates.
- Purchase toys made from fabric, wood or metal (not lead).
- Buy phthalate-free cosmetics, nail polish and other beauty products. See *www.ewg.org* "Skin Deep: Cosmetic Safety Database".
- Buy phthalate-free detergents and other household cleaning products.

### *Dioxin*

Dioxins are released into the air after the incineration of PVC and other waste materials, industrial processes (including smelting), manufacturing of pesticides and herbicides, bleaching of pulp and paper, may be found in tampons, burning household waste and even forest fires. Humans ingest dioxins through the consumption of beef, fish and dairy.

## Tips to Avoid Dioxin

- Use natural paper products and tampons.
- Eat organic whenever possible.
- Avoid high pesticide sprayed foods. See *www.ewg.org* "Dirty Dozen and Clean Fifteen".
- Drink pure, filtered water.

### *Perchlorate*

Ammonium perchlorate is the oxidant in solid rocket fuel. It is also an essential component of military explosives, bottle rockets, fireworks, highway flares, automobile airbags and old-fashioned black powder. Ammonium perchlorate and its other compounds are contaminants of drinking water and some foods such as milk and vegetables.

Research has established that significant amounts of perchlorate disrupt production of thyroid hormones.

## Tips to Avoid Perchlorate

- Drink pure, filtered water.
- Avoid high pesticide sprayed foods. See *www.ewg.org* "Dirty Dozen

and Clean Fifteen".
• Eat organic whenever possible.

## Parabens

Parabens are the most widely used preservative in cosmetics. They are also used as fragrance ingredients. An estimated 75 to 80 % of cosmetics contain parabens.

## Tips to Avoid Parabens
• Read labels of all beauty products and check out *www.ewg.org* "Skin Deep: Cosmetic Safety Database".
• See *www.davidsuzuki.org* "Dirty Dozen Cosmetic Chemicals" for a more extensive list of chemicals to avoid.
• Check out *www.environmentaldefence.ca*

## Progesterone

Progesterone is a steroid hormone that is produced in women by the ovaries during and after ovulation, and during pregnancy, in the placenta. A small amount of progesterone is produced by the adrenal glands. Estrogen dominance often results in a progesterone deficiency, which can lead to common symptoms including:
• Infertility, frequent miscarriages
• PMS, frequent or heavy menstrual periods
• Breast tenderness, fibrocystic breasts
• PCOS
• Increased risk of breast, uterine or ovarian cancer
• Low libido, adrenal fatigue
• Insomnia and anxiety.

## Testosterone

Testosterone is the main male sex hormone, but it is also found in women. It is produced in the ovaries as well as the adrenal glands. Testosterone is a key player in estrogen metabolism. Testosterone converts into estradiol, which plays an important role in maintaining bone mass.

Testosterone also enhances libido, moods, energy, muscle strength and mass and immune function. High levels of testosterone are associated with acne, PCOS, PMS, hair loss on the head, facial hair (on women) and frequent miscarriages.

## *Cortisol*

Cortisol, often called the "stress hormone", is a steroid hormone produced by the adrenal glands (adrenal cortex) in response to stress in order to help the body adapt. High levels of cortisol are associated with increased blood pressure, insomnia, blood sugar and immune system dysfunction among many others. It is also an underlying cause of that dreaded belly fat which starts to accumulate from midlife as a result of the day-to-day stressors and hormonal changes (menopause and andropause) as we age.

## *DHEA*

DHEA is a steroid hormone produced from cholesterol by the adrenal glands, the gonads, adipose tissue and the brain. It serves as a precursor to male and female sex hormones (androgens and estrogens). Low DHEA can cause fatigue, low memory, decreased libido, anxiety, elevated blood pressure, high cholesterol, atherosclerosis, increased infections and poor recovery from stress.

## *Thyroid Hormones*

Thyroid stimulating hormone (TSH) is secreted by the pituitary gland in the brain and causes the thyroid to release thyroid hormones (T3 and T4). TSH is the blood test of choice by most conventional medical doctors and it is considered "normal" if the TSH falls within the reference range (0.4 - 5.0 IU/ml). However, naturopathic doctors and complementary health care professionals are using a new "norm" for the TSH lab value between 0.4 and 2.5 IU/ml and will treat for hypothyroidism if the individual has accompanying symptoms.

Low thyroid hormones can cause a variety of symptoms - to learn more read the **Hypothyroidism** Chapter.

## Aldosterone

Aldosterone is a steroid hormone produced by the adrenal glands (adrenal cortex) and acts on the kidneys to cause the conservation of sodium, secretion of potassium, increased water retention, and increased blood pressure. If salt levels in the body are low, aldosterone signals the kidneys to reabsorb and retain salt thereby retaining water.

## Insulin

Insulin is a hormone produced by the pancreas, which is essential for regulating carbohydrate and fat metabolism in the body. Insulin causes the cells in the liver, muscle and fat tissue to take up glucose from the blood, storing it as glycogen in the liver and muscle. Poor diet and the consumption of high glycemic and refined foods cause increased levels of sugar (glucose) in the body, which signals the release of insulin. Chronically high levels of glucose cause the release of vast amounts of insulin. If this continues over time, the insulin receptors become resistant and do not recognize the hormone any more. Insulin resistance is associated with PCOS, diabetes, PMS, low thyroid disease, and cardiovascular disease.

## Insulin-like Growth Factor (IGF-1)

Insulin-like growth factor (IGF-1) has a molecular structure similar to insulin and is made and secreted primarily in the liver. It helps regulate the cycle of cell growth, division and death. Elevated levels of IGF-1 are associated with increased tissue growth and may promote growth and invasiveness of malignant cells. This may increase the risk of certain cancers (breast, lung, uterine, ovarian) as well as PCOS, fibroids, and ovarian cysts.

## Prolactin

Prolactin, a hormone secreted by the pituitary gland, stimulates lactation (milk production). Abnormally high levels of prolactin can delay puberty, interfere with ovulation in women, cause PCOS and decrease fertility. High prolactin levels can be due to estrogen dominance, low thyroid, stress, hypoglycemia and pregnancy.

## *Melatonin*

Melatonin is a hormone released by the pineal gland in the brain and involved in regulating sleep/wake cycles. Low levels of melatonin are associated with insomnia, fatigue in the morning, morning anxiety, and estrogen dominance. Because of its connection with estrogen dominance, low melatonin can increase the risk of uterine fibroids, uterine and breast cancer. Recent research connects low melatonin with prostate cancer and melanoma.

## *Growth Hormone*

Growth hormone is made in the pituitary gland and stimulates the release of somatomedin by the liver, thereby causing growth. High levels of growth hormone are caused by stress and estrogen dominance, which can increase the risk of PCOS and estrogen dominant conditions including breast cancer, uterine fibroids, ovarian cancer and cysts.

——————— CHAPTER 2 ———————

# ADRENAL FATIGUE

It is surprising how many people have never heard of the adrenal glands, considering they command the most powerful hormones which affect virtually every system in the body. The adrenal glands are no bigger than a walnut and sit on top of each kidney. You cannot live without your adrenal glands and their hormones. How well your adrenal glands function greatly influences your quality of life and vitality.

The hormones secreted by your adrenal glands influence all major physiological processes in the body: utilization of carbohydrates, fats and proteins; regulation of blood sugar; functioning of the cardiovascular, gastrointestinal, immune and nervous systems; inflammation and allergic reactions; hormonal health and more.

Each adrenal gland consists of two parts - the cortex and the medulla. The adrenal cortex secretes a variety of steroid hormones: glucocorticoids (cortisol), mineralocorticoids (aldosterone) and androgens (testosterone). The glucocorticoids affect blood sugar levels. Mineralocorticoids have an effect on mineral metabolism and maintenance of healthy blood pressure. The adrenal cortex also secretes precursor hormones to androgens such as testosterone and other steroid hormones.

The inner part, the adrenal medulla, consists of a group of hormones called catecholamines (epinephrine and norepinephrine also known as adrenaline and noradrenaline). These hormones are released in response to physical or mental stress, known as our "fight or flight" response. During the fight or flight response, the heart pumps harder increasing blood pressure and heart rate. There is an increased demand for energy so blood sugar levels rise as well. Blood flows to the brain; lungs, muscles and cardiac output are all affected, as the body prepares to protect itself from imminent danger.

Unfortunately, in our society, we have too much chronic stress so the *relaxation response* (where blood pressure, digestive function, heart rate, and hormonal levels return to their normal state) doesn't kick in. Lives are too busy, expectations are too high, and bills need to be paid whether you have the money in the bank right now or not. This constant stress causes sustained cortisol output, which is linked to blood sugar problems, fat accumulation, compromised immune function, exhaustion, bone loss, and even heart disease. Memory loss has even been associated with high cortisol levels.

Over time, sustained high cortisol output can cause adrenal gland exhaustion, linked to Chronic Fatigue Syndrome and, in some cases, Addison's disease. As we'll see time and again throughout this book, our hormones work together in a well-rehearsed symphony. Problems with one undoubtedly will affect others, and this is true for the adrenal gland hormones. The adrenals are intimately connected with thyroid function, and compromised adrenal gland output is sure to affect thyroid function (see **Hypothyroidism** Chapter).

**FACT - Did You Know?**

There are less obvious stressors that can affect healthy adrenal gland function. Some examples include:

- Trauma: car accidents, surgery, root canal, death of a loved one
- Nutritional: caffeine, sugar, alcohol, processed/junk foods
- Electromagnetic: cell phones, computers, microwaves, TV
- Environmental: heavy metals, hormones, pesticides and other pollutants, both legal and illicit drugs.

## How Do The Adrenal Glands Fit Into The Hormonal Picture?

Your adrenal glands play an important role in how you experience peri-menopause and menopause. Peri-menopause is the gradual cessation of menstrual periods. It accompanies a roller coaster of hormone activity, with estrogen and progesterone rising and falling – potentially triggering the telltale symptoms of hot flashes, night sweats, headaches and mood swings (see **Menopause** Chapter). One of the main roles of progesterone is to balance the unwanted effects of excess estrogen. Unfortunately, the stress hormone cortisol competes for, and blocks progesterone receptors, meaning that progesterone can't do what it's supposed to do. During chronic stress, progesterone is also converted into the stress hormone cortisol to help the body adapt to stress, rather than converting to estrogens and testosterone in the steroid pathway. This "progesterone steal" causes a shift in hormone production, which leads to a decreased production of estrogen, testosterone, progesterone and DHEA.

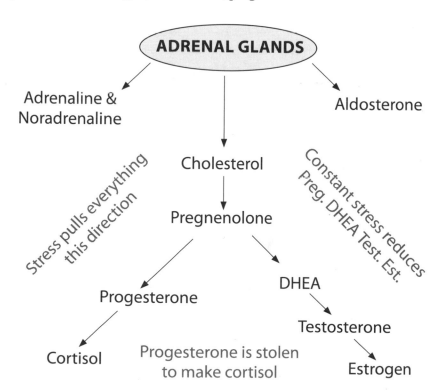

It's crucial to note that progesterone is manufactured not only in the ovaries during ovulation, but also in smaller amounts by the adrenal glands. This becomes particularly important in the 10-15 years before menopause when women may have anovulatory cycles (without ovulation), because it is ovulation that triggers the production of progesterone. When ovulation doesn't occur, the adrenal glands are meant to take over progesterone production. The same story holds true for estrogen. Although this hormone is typically manufactured in the reproductive organs, it's also created by the adrenal glands. When reproduction shuts down at menopause, women still need some estrogen, and the responsibility for making it falls to the adrenal glands. If the adrenal glands are exhausted, they can't create all the hormones you need.

## SIGNS and SYMPTOMS

Adrenal fatigue stretches from mild to severe forms and is caused by some form of acute stress or ongoing chronic stress. The stressors are varied – ranging from emotional, financial, psychological, environmental and infectious or a combination of these over a period of time. Adrenal fatigue occurs when the adrenal glands are no longer able to adapt to the amount of stress encountered by the body.

One of the most common symptoms and usually one of the first symptoms to appear is low energy. Initially, some individuals with adrenal fatigue may appear quite normal but live with a feeling of always having to push themselves or use stimulants in the form of caffeine or sugar to keep them going.

The following "Adrenal Stress Indicator" questionnaire is used by many naturopathic doctors in determining the status of adrenal gland health and function. See how you score!

## ADRENAL STRESS INDICATOR

Write the number "1" beside symptoms you have had in the past; "2" beside symptoms that occur occasionally; "3" beside symptoms that occur often; "4" beside symptoms that occur frequently. Add up the total score.

- ( ) Blurred vision/spots in front of eyes
- ( ) Hormonal imbalances (i.e. thyroid problems)
- ( ) History of asthma/bronchitis
- ( ) Prolonged exposure to stress (job, family, illness, caregiving)
- ( ) Headaches
- ( ) Environmental or chemical exposure or sensitivities
- ( ) Hypoglycemia/blood sugar problems – Mood swings
- ( ) Food allergies
- ( ) Poor concentration/memory problems (Alzheimer's disease)
- ( ) Low energy, excessive fatigue
- ( ) Easily overwhelmed, inability to handle stress
- ( ) Post-exertion fatigue
- ( ) Dizziness upon standing (or fainting)
- ( ) Inflammatory conditions (Arthritis, bursitis)
- ( ) Nervousness/anxiety, depression, irritability or anger
- ( ) Shortness of breath/yawning (air hunger)
- ( ) Cold hands or feet
- ( ) Low back pain, knee problems, sore muscles
- ( ) Insomnia/frequent waking
- ( ) Excessive urination
- ( ) Excessive perspiration or no perspiration
- ( ) Heart palpitations
- ( ) Edema of extremities or general edema
- ( ) Eyes light-sensitive
- ( ) Cravings: sugar, salt or coffee and other stimulants
- ( ) Alcohol intolerance
- ( ) Recurrent colds or infections
- ( ) Digestive problems, ulcers
- ( ) Weight gain or weight loss
- ( ) High or low blood pressure
- ( ) **Total Score**

## If you scored...

- Between 30 and 50, you've received an early-warning indicator that your adrenals are starting to weaken.
- Between 50 and 80 – start with adrenal support such as **AdrenaSense®**.
- Between 80 and 100 – your adrenal glands are taxed so you might want to take an adrenal glandular with your **AdrenaSense®**.
- Over 100 – you are suffering from adrenal exhaustion and will require long-term adrenal support.

Common diseases or conditions associated with stress and adrenal fatigue:

- Metabolic Syndrome and Diabetes
- Obesity
- Cardiovascular disease
- Anxiety disorders and depression
- Immune compromise and some cancers
- Allergies and chemical sensitivities
- Inflammatory disorders (arthritis)
- Hormonal imbalances (i.e. polycystic ovary syndrome)
- Osteoporosis
- Alzheimer's disease and memory loss
- Insomnia
- Chronic Fatigue Syndrome/Fibromyalgia
- Asthma and bronchitis
- Gastrointestinal disorders (colitis).

## DIAGNOSIS

Unfortunately, most individuals who suffer from adrenal fatigue are often missed or misdiagnosed by conventional medicine, even though the individual may exhibit all of the classic symptoms.

Today, modern medicine relies strictly on clinical testing to diagnose conditions. Although clear lab testing is absolutely necessary for a diagnosis, it misses the people who may be in the earlier stages of the disease. Even pre-clinical stages of a disease can have debilitating symptoms associated with it. There are tests, however usually performed by naturopathic doctors or complementary health care providers to assess adrenal function. These tests include:

- **Saliva Adrenal Profile Testing** – Saliva hormone testing measures the amounts of various stress hormones in the saliva instead of blood or urine. Saliva measures the amount of hormone inside the cells, whereas blood measures hormones outside the cells.

- **Ragland effect – Postural Hypotension** – Normally, when a person goes from the lying position to standing, the systolic blood pressure should elevate 5-10 mm Hg (millimeters of mercury). In adrenal fatigue, the systolic blood pressure from lying to standing will either drop or stay the same. Assessing the blood pressure change can help determine the level of adrenal fatigue.

- **Pupillary Response** – Adrenal fatigue will cause an imbalance between sodium and potassium. One of the signs of this electrolyte imbalance is the pupillary reflex. Shining a light into a person's eye should cause the pupil to constrict and remain constricted for 30 seconds. In the adrenal-fatigued individual, especially in the later stages, the pupil will fluctuate open and closed in response to the light. Or the pupil will initially constrict but dilate again in less than 30 seconds – even with continued light.

- **Koenisberg Test** – This is a urinary test that measures chloride and gives an indirect measurement of sodium and potassium excretion. Many Naturopathic doctors use this test in their clinics.

- **Medical History** - The Naturopathic doctor must also do a thorough history, looking at all stressful events including: surgeries and hospital stays; illnesses such as a bad bout of the flu, pneumonia, long term pain, dental work such as a root canal or implants; emotional stress such as job loss, moving, death of a friend or relative, divorce, financial problems and other stressful events.

## PREVENTION and TREATMENT – Dietary and Lifestyle

### FOOD FACTORS

The most important change you can make to support your adrenal glands is to remove unhealthy coping strategies from your life. Cigarettes, alcohol and poor diet are detrimental in so many ways, but when you're stressed your body uses up more vitamins and minerals. Therefore, it's crucial that you have them in your diet in ample supply – and you're not going to get them in your drive-through hamburger combo! Enjoy a balanced diet including plenty of fresh, raw fruit and vegetables, whole grains and lean protein. Organic produce is best, as pesticides, herbicides and fungicides stress the liver – which in turn stresses your adrenals. Be sure your diet includes plenty of vitamin C foods (peppers, tomatoes, citrus), magnesium (pumpkin seeds, spinach, oat bran, almonds), zinc (sesame seeds, pumpkin seeds, venison) and B complex vitamins (leafy greens, egg yolk, fish, whole grains), which are key adrenal boosting vitamins. Build a strong foundation for your health with a daily multi-vitamin/multi-mineral supplement, along with omega-3 essential fatty acids to reduce inflammation and promote mental calmness. Stay away from caffeine. Although you might think it calms you, caffeine actually increases cortisol levels. Instead, enjoy herbal teas containing adaptogens like ashwagandha, schizandra berries, astragalus, hawthorn berries and lemongrass to promote energy.

### LIFESTYLE TIPS

- The key to supporting adrenal recovery is to learn how to promote the relaxation response several times a day. While this might seem more stressful as you add to your 'to do' list, some relaxation strategies are as simple as stopping to take a deep breath. Along with helping to bring a sense of calm, deep breathing also releases endorphins (the body's natural pain killers) and relaxes muscles. Try this exercise while seated at your desk, stuck in traffic, waiting through soccer practice or while watching television:

> *Sit up straight in your chair.*
> *Exhale through pursed lips.*
> *Inhale through your nose, and relax the belly muscles.*
> *Draw your breath down into your belly.*
> *After your belly is full, continue to inhale, and fill up your chest.*
> *Feel your rib cage expand.*
> *Hold the breath for a moment, then exhale very slowly.*
> *Relax your chest and rib cage.*
> *Pull in your belly to expend the remaining breath.*
> *Repeat for about five minutes.*

- Other techniques to promote relaxation include meditation, journaling, yoga, sex, singing at the top of your lungs in the car or in the shower, or regularly renting a comedy. Perhaps the most beneficial stress-alleviating technique is moderate exercise. This one makes a lot of sense. When our ancestors were startled by a sabre-toothed lion, they either ran or fought. Both activities would 'burn off' the stress hormones and allow your body to eventually move into the relaxation response. Exercise also cuts down on cigarette cravings if you are using stress as a dangerous excuse to smoke.

- Because you don't want to be stressed and cranky, aim for eight hours of sleep each night. In circular fashion, research also suggests that inadequate sleep can increase cortisol levels. Turn off the television or computer at least a few hours before bed as looking at screens diminishes your ability to relax. Instead, light some candles and listen to soft music as you enjoy a relaxing Epsom salt bath.

- Use adaptogenic herbs to support adrenal glands. Quite simply, adaptogens help your body adapt to stress by enhancing energy, improving mental calmness and clarity or improving sleep.

## KEY SUPPLEMENTS

Rhodiola - *Rhodiola rosea*
Rhodiola rosea has been studied extensively and has been categorized as an adaptogenic herb by Russian researchers for its ability to increase resistance in the body to a variety of chemical, biological and physical stressors. This anti-stress herb has a reputation for stimulating the nervous system, eliminating fatigue, enhancing work performance, and decreasing depression. It has been shown to prevent stress-induced catecholamine over-release in cardiac tissue thus helping to protect the cardiopulmonary system. Rhodiola also has anti-cancer, anti-aging properties and may help with high altitude sickness.

DOSAGE: *100–500 mg daily*

Suma - *Pfaffia paniculata*
Suma has been traditionally used in Brazil as an energy and rejuvenating tonic, as well as a general cure-all for many disorders. It is excellent for the cardiovascular system, central nervous system, reproductive, digestive and immune systems.

DOSAGE: *100 mg one to three times daily*

### Body/Mind Connection

Adrenal fatigue is linked with anxiety and not taking care of yourself. Focus on loving yourself and self-care.

Ashwagandha - *Withania somnifera*
Ashwagandha is an important herb in Ayurvedic medicine. It serves as an adaptogen helping the adrenal glands combat stress as well as supports healthy thyroid function by supporting the synthesis of thyroid hormones.

DOSAGE: *300–1000 mg daily*

## Siberian Ginseng - *Eleutherococcus senticosus*

Siberian Ginseng has been studied extensively for its adaptogenic and anti-stress properties. Data indicates that it increases the ability to accommodate to adverse physical conditions, improves mental performance, and enhances the quality of work under stressful conditions. Eleutherococcus has been studied extensively (more than 1,000 papers have been published over the last three decades on Eleutherococcus) and has a long and continued history of use in Siberia and China to increase the length and quality of life, prevent infection, improve memory and improve appetite. It has a bitter-warming and sweet-warming quality. Compared to Panax ginseng, Eleutherococcus is less stimulating, tends to have a more rapid action and has a more generalized effect on immunity.

DOSAGE: *100 mg one to four times daily*

## Schizandra berries - *Schizandra chinensis*

Schizandra chinensis, a member of the Magnoliaceae family, has an extensive history of medical use in China. This herb's adaptogenic properties increase resistance to a wide range of physical, chemical, and emotional stresses while promoting improved overall regulation of physiological processes. Experimental evidence suggests Schizandra has liver protective abilities and functions as a potent antioxidant.

DOSAGE: *100 mg one to four times daily*

*\*\*\*All the above herbs are found in **AdrenaSense®**, an excellent product for supporting healthy adrenal function and combating symptoms of adrenal fatigue and stress.*

## Flaxseed Oil and/or Pure Fish Oil - Omega-3 Fatty Acids

Essential fatty acids, specifically omega-3s in the form of flaxseed or uncontaminated fish oil, decrease the formation of PGE2 - a messenger molecule that promotes inflammatory pathways in the body. By decreasing inflammation, the overall stress on the body is reduced thus helping to support optimal adrenal function. Omegas-3s also help support healthy cardiovascular and nervous systems.

DOSAGE: *Take up to 2 tbsp of flax oil daily and/or up to 3000 mg fish oil daily with a minimum of 800 EPA and 400 mg DHA.*

## B Vitamins

### Vitamin B6 - Pyridoxine and P5P
Vitamin B6 is a necessary cofactor for the formation of several important neurotransmitters such as GABA, serotonin and dopamine, which are commonly associated with stress.

DOSAGE: *100–250 mg daily*

### Vitamin B5 - Pantothenic acid
Vitamin B5 is an important B vitamin for supporting the adrenal cortex and regulating cortisol levels during periods of high stress.

DOSAGE: *100–500 mg daily*

### Vitamin B12 - Methylcobalamin
Stress often disrupts the body's natural circadian rhythmic secretion of cortisol. This disruption in cortisol levels can greatly interfere with melatonin production and lead to insomnia and other problems with sleep. Vitamin B12 is thought to have an effect on helping to reset healthy secretion of cortisol during periods of stress thus improving the stress response and quality of sleep.

DOSAGE: *1000–5000 mcg daily*

### Folic Acid - 5-Methyltetrahydrofolate
Folic acid is an important co-factor in the formation of serotonin, dopa-

mine, norepinephrine and epinephrine and therefore essential for supporting healthy adrenal gland function and the stress response.

DOSAGE: *1–5 mg daily*

## Vitamin C

Vitamin C is very important because it is used in the formation of adrenal hormones such as cortisol. During times of stress, the body's requirement for vitamin C can increase 10- to 20-fold.

DOSAGE: *1–3 grams daily or to bowel tolerance*

## Magnesium bisglycinate

Magnesium is important for energy production of every cell in the body and essential for adrenal gland recovery.

DOSAGE: *200–800 mg daily*

*\*Note: some magnesium such as magnesium oxide or magnesium citrate can cause diarrhea even at low doses in some people, so adjust dosage to your own optimal level.*

## GABA - gamma-Aminobutyric Acid

GABA is a major neurotransmitter widely distributed throughout the central nervous system. Too much excitation can lead to irritability, restlessness, insomnia, seizures, and movement disorders. This must be balanced with inhibition. GABA is the most important inhibitory neurotransmitter in the brain and acts like a "break" during times of runaway stress and brain excitability. This supplement is ideal for those individuals who cannot "turn off their brain".

DOSAGE: *100–500 mg daily*

## L-Tyrosine

Findings from several studies suggest supplementation with tyrosine will reduce the acute effects of stress and fatigue on task performance. Stress depletes the brain reserves of the catecholamine neurotransmitters norepinephrine and dopamine; and it appears that this depletion, especially of norepinephrine, is closely related to stress-induced performance decline. Administration of tyrosine, an amino acid precursor of the above catecholamines, therefore alleviates both the depletion of brain catecholamines and the stress-induced decline in performance.

DOSAGE: *100–500 mg daily*

## 5-HTP – 5-Hydroxytryptophan

5-Hydroxytryptophan acts primarily by increasing CNS levels of serotonin, our "happy hormone". Serotonin levels greatly determine our moods, sleep and general well-being. Other neurotransmitters and CNS chemicals, such as melatonin, dopamine, norepinephrine, and beta-endorphin, have also been shown to increase following oral administration of 5-HTP. During times of stress, the above neurotransmitters are depleted and therefore supplementation with 5-HTP may be beneficial.

DOSAGE: *100–200 mg two to three times daily*

## Zinc

Zinc is an essential mineral for immune function as well as supporting healthy adrenal function.

DOSAGE: *10–50 mg daily with food*

## L-Theanine

L-theanine is an amino acid extracted from green or black tea. In the brain, L-theanine increases dopamine, serotonin, and the inhibitory neurotransmitter glycine. Studies show that L-theanine can induce a perceived state of relaxation in an individual while staying alert.

DOSAGE: *100–300 mg daily*

## Maca – *Lepidium meyeii*

Maca is a root vegetable cultivated in the Peruvian Andes that belongs to the brassica (mustard) family. Maca is rich in amino acids, iodine, iron, and magnesium. Maca increases energy and may be useful for supporting the body's stress response and healthy adrenal function.

DOSAGE: *2–4 capsules daily of* **Ultimate Maca Energy™**, *1 tsp daily of* **Maca-Punch Platinum Liquid Extract™** *or 1 tbsp of* **Ultimate Maca Energy Powder™**

## Probiotics – *Lactobacillus acidophilus and Bifidobacterium spp.*

Stress has a significant influence on intestinal microflora. Chronic stress will upset the balance between "good" bacteria and "bad" bacteria.

DOSAGE: *at least 10 billion CFU daily with food.*

## CONVENTIONAL MEDICINE

Conventional medicine typically does not recognize adrenal fatigue or exhaustion because conventional lab testing only identifies the most extreme adrenal diseases such as Addison's and Cushing's disease. This often misses those individuals who may be in the earlier stages of the disease. The pre-clinical stages of a disease can have debilitating symptoms associated with it, but patients are told that there is nothing wrong and that their problems are "all in their head" because all lab tests come back within "normal" range.

Addison's disease is at the extreme low end of adrenal function and is life threatening if left untreated. Patients are usually prescribed corticosteroid hormones for the rest of their lives.

Cushing's syndrome is the extreme high end of adrenal function caused by prolonged exposure to the stress hormone cortisol. Medications may be prescribed to control excessive production of cortisol secreted from the adrenal glands or surgery may be suggested if the cause is a tumour on the pituitary or adrenal gland.

—————— CHAPTER 3 ——————

# BIRTH CONTROL

For many couples, choosing a method of birth control that is effective and mutually satisfying can be difficult. Women should discuss all options with their naturopathic doctor or medical professional to determine the effectiveness, health benefits and health risks of each contraceptive method. A summary of pros and cons of birth control methods is outlined below.

## Abstinence

This is defined as not having sex <u>at any time</u>.

***Pros:***
- 100% effective

***Cons:***
- No intercourse

## Withdrawal/Pull-out Method

This is a method of birth control in which a man, during intercourse withdraws prior to ejaculation.

***Pros:***
- 77-85% effective

## Cons:

- Requires a great deal of control
- Leakage of sperm may occur before ejaculation
- May decrease sexual fulfillment
- Success is determined by male partner.

## Fertility Awareness/Rhythm Method/Natural Family Planning

Many couples use this method to try to determine a woman's fertile period as well as when to abstain from having intercourse to prevent pregnancy. Couples do not have intercourse or use a barrier method on the days that a woman is most fertile.

Most women have a menstrual cycle every 26 to 32 days with ovulation occurring on Day 14 – Mid-cycle. Intercourse should be avoided at least three days before and three days after ovulation, typically Day 11 through to Day 17. A woman is often most fertile 48 hours before ovulation and within 24 hours after ovulation.

It is helpful if the woman's cycle is regular or charting can become difficult.

Cervical mucous can be used to predict ovulation. Its appearance resembles egg white.

Basal body temperature is also used to predict ovulation by measuring one's temperature under the arm or orally first thing in the morning before getting out of bed. The body temperature may drop slightly (usually around half a degree) just before ovulation, and then goes up approximately one degree from there just after ovulation and remains steady until menses. If the temperature remains high longer than the expected 12 to 14 days then pregnancy is usually indicated.

## Pros:

- 90% effective
- Avoids drugs, hormones, chemicals and their unwanted side effects
- No cost
- Woman develops awareness of her own cycle.

*Cons:*
- Does not protect against sexually transmitted diseases (STDs)
- Requires a high degree of discipline for it to work
- Needs to be combined with barrier methods on fertile days
- Involves acceptance by sexual partner.

*Some Precautions:*
- Woman's menstrual cycle needs to be regular – cycles may shift due to stress, sickness, travel, diet, and exercise.

## Condom

A male condom is a thin sheath placed over the erect penis and left in place during sexual intercourse. Using condoms with an intravaginal spermicide can provide more protection and is the preferred method for some couples.

*Pros:*
- 88-98% effective
- Inexpensive and easy to use
- Best method for STD protection
- Good results when used with spermicide.

*Cons:*
- Condoms may break
- Reliance on male partner
- May reduce sensation and spontaneity.

*Some Precautions:*
- Condoms can be irritating to some women especially if there is a latex allergy. If this occurs, condoms made from lambskin can be used.

## Female Condom

This is a type of barrier method using a device inserted into the vagina before intercourse. The female condom is a soft, loose-fitting polyurethane pouch with a ring on each end. Before intercourse, one ring is inserted into the vagina to hold the female condom in place. The ring at the open end of the condom remains outside the vagina covering the labia.

### Pros:
- 95% effective
- Protects against STDs
- Can be inserted up to eight hours before intercourse
- Does not need to be removed immediately after intercourse
- Decreases the risk of cervical dysplasia
- Woman is in control
- No need for a prescription or special fitting.

### Cons:
- Can only be used once
- Need to practice insertion to become comfortable with device
- Condom can break.

### Some Precautions:
- During intercourse, the female condom may slip out of the vagina. The couple must be sure that the penis enters the female condom properly and does not slip between the vagina and the outside of the female condom. Sometimes the outer ring of the female condom gets pushed into the vagina during intercourse.

## Diaphragm with Spermicide

The diaphragm is a contraceptive device that prevents sperm from entering the uterus. It is a small, reusable rubber or silicone cup with a flexible rim that covers the cervix. Before sexual intercourse, the diaphragm is inserted deep into the vagina so part of the rim fits snugly behind the pubic bone. The diaphragm is held in place by the vaginal muscles. It must be fitted and prescribed by a medical professional. Spermicide is applied on the diaphragm before insertion and the device is left in place for at least six hours after intercourse.

### Pros:
- 82-94% effective

- Inexpensive
- Can be inserted up to six hours before intercourse.

**Cons:**
- Must be initially fitted by a medical professional
- Must leave in for at least six hours after intercourse
- Reapplication of spermicide necessary for repeated intercourse DO NOT REMOVE THE DIAPHRAGM – Insert spermicide into vagina with an applicator
- Can increase risk of urinary tract infections
- Does not protect against STDs
- May be uncomfortable
- Practice insertion to become comfortable with device.

**Some Precautions:**
- Your health care provider may discourage the use of a diaphragm if you have an allergy to silicone, latex or spermicide; have vaginal abnormalities that interfere with the fit, placement or retention of the diaphragm; have frequent urinary tract infections; or have uterine prolapse.

## Cervical Cap with Spermicide

The cervical cap is a contraceptive device that prevents sperm from entering the uterus. It is a reusable, deep cup that fits tightly over the cervix. Before sexual intercourse, the cervical cap is inserted into the vagina. The cervical cap is held in place by suction and has a strap to help with removal. The cervical cap is effective at preventing pregnancy only when used with spermicide.

**Pros:**
- 82-94% effective
- Can be inserted 30 minutes to 48 hours before sexual intercourse
- Inexpensive
- Good for women who have frequent intercourse as it can be left in for 48 hours.

**Cons:**

- Must leave in for six to eight hours after intercourse
- Increased risk of changes in cervical cells
- May cause discomfort upon insertion
- Does not protect against STDs
- May cause vaginal discharge or odour if left in too long
- May be difficult to insert
- Risk of toxic shock syndrome if cap is left in for longer than 48 hours.

**Some Precautions:**

- Your health care provider may discourage the use of the cervical cap if you have an allergy to spermicide or silicone; have a history of pelvic inflammatory disease, toxic shock syndrome, cervical cancer, uterine tract infections or vaginal or cervical tissue tears; or have a vaginal abnormality.

## The Contraceptive Sponge

The contraceptive sponge is a contraceptive device that prevents sperm from entering the uterus. It is a soft, disk-shaped device made of polyurethane foam that covers the cervix. Before sexual intercourse, the sponge is inserted deep into the vagina and held in place by vaginal muscles. The contraceptive sponge has a strap to assist with removal and contains spermicide, which blocks or kills sperm.

**Pros:**

- 72-94% effective
- Insertion up to 24 hours before intercourse
- No need for reapplication of spermicide for repeated intercourse
- Easily obtained.

**Cons:**

- May cause vaginal dryness
- May be uncomfortable
- Does not protect against STDs.

## Intrauterine Devices – Copper IUD

The copper IUD is a small, soft flexible device containing copper that is inserted into the uterus for long-term contraception. The T-shaped plastic frame continuously releases copper and prevents sperm from entering the fallopian tubes and fertilizing the egg.

### Pros:

- 97-99% effective
- Lasts up to ten years
- Effective upon insertion
- Reversible – can be removed at any time
- No need for planning or remembering
- Does not carry the risk of side effects related to hormone releasing forms of birth control.

### Cons:

- Increased risk of pelvic inflammatory disease and ectopic pregnancy
- May cause increased cramping and bleeding
- Must be inserted by a medical professional
- No protection from STDs
- May perforate uterus or be expelled.

### Some Precautions:

- The copper IUD should not be used by women who have a: history of pelvic inflammatory disease, copper allergy or Wilson's disease, history of ectopic pregnancy, or abnormal uterine anatomy.

### Side Effects:

- Cramps, severe menstrual pain and heavy bleeding, breakthrough bleeding, nausea, anemia, backache, painful sex, inflammation of the vagina, vaginal discharge or an itchy rash.

## Intrauterine Devices – Progestin IUD (Mirena)

Mirena is a hormonal intrauterine device (IUD) that's inserted into the uterus for long-term contraception. The T-shaped plastic frame releases the hormone progestin, which thickens the cervical mucous and thins the lining of the uterus (endometrium) - preventing sperm from entering the fallopian tubes. Mirena also partially suppresses ovulation and can prevent pregnancy for up to five years after insertion.

**Pros:**
- 97-99% effective
- Lasts up to five years
- Effective upon insertion
- Reversible – can be removed at any time
- No need for planning or remembering.

**Cons:**
- Increased risk of pelvic inflammatory disease and ectopic pregnancy
- May cause increased cramping and bleeding
- Must be inserted by a medical professional
- No protection from STDs
- May perforate uterus or be expelled
- Exposure to synthetic progestin long term.

**Some Precautions:**
- Mirena should not be used by women who have a history of breast cancer; have uterine, cervical or liver cancer; have uterine abnormalities, such as fibroids; have a pelvic infection or history of pelvic inflammatory disease; or have an abnormal pap smear.

**Side Effects:**
- Headaches, acne, breast tenderness, breakthrough bleeding, absence of periods, mood changes, weight gain, nausea, ovarian cysts, abdominal or pelvic pain.

## Birth Control Pill

The birth control pill is a combination of synthetic estrogen and progestin. It is taken daily to prevent the ovaries from releasing an egg. It can also cause changes in the lining of the uterus and the cervical mucous to keep the sperm from joining the egg.

**Pros:**
- 99% effective

- Continuous protection when taken correctly
- Decreases menstrual cramps and improves hormonal acne.

**Cons:**
- Must be remembered/taken daily
- Increased risk of blood clots, heart attack, stroke, especially in smokers over age 35
- Increased breast and liver cancer risk
- Increased cervical dysplasia
- Does not protect against STDs.

**Side Effects:**
- Depression, mood swings, nausea, migraines, yeast and chlamydia infections, breast tenderness, lowered libido, bloating, breakthrough bleeding. More serious: hair loss, blood clots, high blood pressure, heart attack and elevated liver enzymes.

**Vitamin and Mineral Deficiencies:**
- The birth control pill depletes the following vitamins and minerals: B vitamins especially B6, B1, B2, B3, B12, folic acid, zinc, vitamin C, magnesium and selenium.

## Depo-Provera

Depo-Provera is a well-known brand name for medroxyprogesterone acetate, a contraceptive injection for women that contains the synthetic hormone progestin. Depo-Provera is given as an injection once every three months and works by suppressing ovulation and keeping the ovaries from releasing an egg. Depo-Provera also thickens cervical mucous to keep sperm from reaching the egg.

**Pros:**
- Over 99% effective
- No need to remember to take a daily pill
- Mostly reversible – fertility returns in 70% of women within one year of stopping injections
- Lowers risk of endometrial cancer
- Continuous protection for up to five years.

## Cons:

- Must visit medical professional every three months for injection
- Delayed return to fertility (5-18 months)
- Increased breast cancer risk
- Completely suppresses menstruation after one year of use and can take one year for fertility to return
- Decreased bone mineral density after one injection
- May cause diabetes.

## Some Precautions:

- Depo-Provera should not be used by women who have a history of blood clotting problems, risk factors for osteoporosis, liver disease, breast cancer or unexplained vaginal bleeding.

## Side Effects:

- Abdominal pain, acne, breast soreness, depression, headaches, irregular periods or breakthrough bleeding, loss of bone mineral density, nervousness, weakness and fatigue, weight gain, stimulates appetite, irritability and risk of diabetes.

## Tubal Ligation

Tubal ligation, also known as "having your tubes tied", is a surgical procedure in which the fallopian tubes are closed by being cut, tied, or sealed to permanently prevent pregnancy. This stops the eggs from travelling down to the uterus where they can be fertilized and blocks the sperm from traveling up the fallopian tubes to the egg. A tubal ligation does not affect a woman's menstrual cycle. Sometimes, a woman having cesarean birth has the procedure done at the same time, so as to avoid having additional surgery later. Tubal ligation is reversible, however, major surgery is required and is not always effective.

## Pros:

- Over 99% effective
- Continuous contraceptive protection
- No need to remember daily.

**Cons:**
- Permanent, although can be reversed through surgery but not always effective
- Surgery may cause increased cramping, irregular periods or heavier bleeding
- Does not protect from STDs.

**Some Precautions:**
- Since tubal ligation is a surgical procedure some risks associated include damage to the bowel, bladder or major blood vessels, poor wound healing or risk of infection or prolonged pelvic or abdominal pain.

## Male Vasectomy

A vasectomy is a form of male birth control that cuts and seals the tubes that carry sperm. It is generally straightforward and is low risk. A vasectomy is considered a permanent form of male birth control and therefore an individual or couples should be certain that they don't want any children in the future.

**Pros:**
- Over 99% effective
- Continuous contraceptive protection
- No need to remember daily.

**Cons:**
- Considered permanent (very difficult to reverse)
- Invasive surgery
- Does not protect against STDs.

**Some Precautions:**
- For most men, a vasectomy does not cause any noticeable side effects, and serious complications are rare. Some side effects right after surgery may include swelling, bruising of the scrotum, bleeding or a blot clot inside the scrotum, blood in the semen, or possible infection.

## KEY SUPPLEMENTS
The birth control pill can lead to many vitamin and mineral deficiencies and therefore it is critical to supplement with the following while taking any oral contraceptives to reduce potential harmful side effects:

Vitamin B6
DOSAGE: *100–200 mg daily*

Folic Acid
DOSAGE: *1–2 mg daily*

Vitamin B12
DOSAGE: *500–1000 mcg daily*

Vitamin B1
DOSAGE: *30 mg daily*

Vitamin B2
DOSAGE: *10 mg daily*

Vitamin B3
DOSAGE: *15 mg daily*

Vitamin C
DOSAGE: *1000–2000 mg daily or to bowel tolerance*

Magnesium
DOSAGE: *150–250 mg daily of magnesium bisglycinate or citrate.*

*\*Note: Magnesium oxide or citrate can cause diarrhea in some individuals, therefore magnesium bisglycinate is the preferred choice because it is more bio-available and better tolerated.*

## Zinc
DOSAGE: *30 mg daily*

## Selenium
DOSAGE: *200 mcg daily*

## Flaxseed Oil and/or Pure Fish Oil – Omega-3 Fatty Acids
Essential fatty acids in the form of flaxseed or uncontaminated fish oil block the formation of PGE2, which is a messenger molecule that helps increase inflammatory pathways in the body. Omega-3 fatty acids also support cardiovascular health, the nervous system and optimal immune functioning.

DOSAGE: *Take up to 2 tbsp of flax oil daily and/or up to 3000 mg fish oil daily with a minimum of 800 mg EPA and 400 mg DHA.*

## Liver Support – *EstroSense*®
Increasing liver detoxification is vitally important to the elimination of harmful estrogens and improving overall health. The birth control pill can put excess stress on the body and the liver through their elimination. Important supplements such as milk thistle, curcumin, indole-3-carbinol, sulforaphane, calcium-d-glucarate, DIM, green tea extract, lycopene, and rosemary extract help support estrogen metabolism through the liver and bind harmful by-products promoting their healthy elimination from the body.

DOSAGE: *3 capsules twice daily*

## Probiotics - *Lactobacillus acidophilus and Bifidobacterium spp.*
Probiotics are known to play an important role in the maintenance of normal flora in the gastrointestinal tract. They also help with the detoxification and binding of harmful estrogens in the digestive tract and eliminate them from the body through the colon. The birth control pill can affect the "good" bacteria in the gut and therefore it may be import-

ant to supplement with probiotics to support a healthy and optimally functioning digestive system.

DOSAGE: *at least 10 billion CFU daily with food.*

CHAPTER 4

# BREAST CANCER

Breast cancer is the most common cancer among Canadian women ages 35 to 54, with an estimated 1 in 9 women developing breast cancer in her lifetime and 1 in 29 who will die from it. With this high statistical risk, especially occurring in the younger population of women, there needs to be a strong focus on breast cancer prevention. According to the Canadian Cancer Society, about 30 to 35% of all cancers can be prevented by eating well, being active and maintaining a healthy body weight. Breast cancers occurring in the mid-thirties age range are usually more aggressive - even more reason for a young woman to adopt preventative measures.

Breast cancer, like cancers in other tissues, begins with changes in the DNA of the breast cell. This can be initiated by a variety of causative agents including genetic, hormonal, physiological and environmental. One of the primary causes of breast cancer is excessive levels of estrogen metabolites. Estrogen is made primarily in the ovaries and is broken down in the liver creating, different forms of estrogen. Some of these estrogens are protective while others can be potentially toxic, leading to different types of estrogen-related cancers.

The female breast consists of 15 to 20 sections called "lobes", each consisting of smaller sections called "lobules". The lobules contain the glands that produce milk. During lactation, breast milk flows from the lobules through tiny tubes called ducts, until eventually it reaches the nipple. Also found in the breast are some of the lymphatic system's lymph vessels, which are connected to lymph nodes. An important part of the body's defense system, lymph nodes create lymphocytes that help to trap debris and foreign particles so they don't enter the blood stream. In reference to breast cancer, lymph nodes are located in the axillary or under-arm area, above the collarbone and behind the breastbone. A younger woman's breast consists mainly of glands and milk ducts, while an older woman's breasts are primarily fatty tissue. Throughout the menstrual cycle, breasts may feel different, often becoming lumpier closer to the time of menstruation. While there are various types of breast cancer, the disease usually starts in the lobules (lobular carcinoma) or most commonly, in the ducts (ductal carcinoma).

Our cells are typically formed, live and die in a preordained way. Sometimes, however, cell replication can go on unchecked, causing a growth that may or may not be cancerous. If DNA is damaged during the replication process, a cell can become abnormal. Typically, the body will find and destroy the abnormal cell, but if the mutated cell is not de-activated, it will continue to replicate itself. This is how cancer begins and cancer's goal is to survive - even at the expense of its host. Cancer will reroute blood supply to steal nutrients. Unlike healthy cells, cancer cells lack pre-programmed cell death (apoptosis). Your best defense against any type of cancer is to minimize your risk and give your body the tools it needs to keep you healthy.

Inheriting the genes linked to breast cancer can account for approximately 5% of cases of the disease. Avoiding other risk factors (listed below), strengthening the immune system and adopting a health-promoting lifestyle are important in preventing breast cancer even if a genetic predisposition exists. Having a mother or sister with breast cancer increases the risk (in the order of 1.5 to 3 times above the average susceptibility risk of 1 in 8) and the older the mother is when diagnosed reduces the risk for the daughter. There is also a greater chance of developing breast cancer if a first, second or third degree relative has been diagnosed with ovarian or endometrial cancer. Women with

BRCA-1 and BRCA-2 gene mutations are more susceptible to both breast and ovarian cancer. Some studies show up to a fourfold increased risk when a brother or father is diagnosed with prostate cancer. While family history plays a role in determining your risk, most women with breast cancer don't have a family history of the disease.

Other known risks include:

- Aging (over age 50)
- Having never given birth or having children after age 30
- Not breastfeeding
- Increased exposure to estrogen caused by hormone replacement therapy (estrogen plus progestin) for more than five years
- Early onset of menstruation (before age 11)
- Late menopause (after age 54)
- Increased breast density
- Overweight or obese after menopause
- Lack of physical activity
- Alcohol consumption
- Cigarette smoking
- Many prescription medications (e.g. Beta- blockers, antidepressants, among others)
- Dental problems (mercury fillings, root canals)
- Chronic inflammation
- Constipation
- Exposure to xenoestrogens (environmental estrogens such as bisphenol-A, phthalates, birth control pills, parabens, hair dyes, non-organic foods sprayed with pesticides and insecticides).

## BREAST CANCER RISK ASSESSMENT

Take the following breast health test and discover if you are at risk for breast cancer.

| | |
|---|---|
| Have not had children and are under 25 years of age | 1 |
| Have not had children and are 25-35 years of age | 1 |
| Have had no children and don't intend to | 3 |
| Did not breastfeed | 2 |
| Had an abortion of the first pregnancy | 1 |
| Took birth control pills during teens or early 20's. A few months use may increase risk by 30% and ten years may double risk. | 3 |
| Taking or have taken HRT (Premarin, Provera, Prempro) | 3 |
| Have had regular mammograms before menopause | 2 |
| Don't exercise three times a week | 2 |
| Have had depression and taking tricyclic anti-depressants | 2 |
| Have breast implants (breast trauma) | 1 |
| Had chest x-rays as a teenager or during 20's | 2 |
| Are exposed to EMFs due to excessive computer use or other | 1 |
| Dye your hair with dark-colored dyes (source of xenoestrogens) | 2 |
| Wear dry-cleaned clothing (source of xenoestrogens) | 1 |
| Use bleached sanitary products e.g. tampons (xenoestrogens) | 2 |
| Eat pesticide and herbicide-laden foods (xenoestrogen source) | 3 |
| Use nail polish remover containing toluene or phthalate | 1 |
| Menstruation started before age of 12 | 2 |
| Late onset menopause after age of 54 | 2 |
| Eat a diet high in animal fat, dairy and meat (xenoestrogens source) | 3 |
| Smoke, started early with excessive use | 3 |
| Alcohol, started early with excessive use | 3 |
| Don't eat cruciferous vegetables (e.g. broccoli, cauliflower, kale) | 3 |
| Take cholesterol-lowering drugs which deplete CoQ10 | 3 |
| Use anti-hypertensives for lowering BP (decreases CoQ10) | 3 |
| Using tranquilizers (studies show increase in breast tumours) | 2 |
| Using ulcer medications which disrupt estrogen metabolism | 2 |
| You are overweight or obese (fat stores estrogens) | 3 |
| Use Flagyl for yeast infections (increases mammary tumours) | 2 |
| Family history in mother, sister or daughter | 1 |

⬭ **Total Score**

**0-18** Lower risk **19-35** Moderate to high risk **35-65** High Risk

## SIGNS and SYMPTOMS – Catch it EARLY!

While the jury still appears to be out on the best form of detection, it's a good idea to be familiar with your own breasts, how they look and feel throughout the month. The National Cancer Institute recommends that you immediately report to your doctor:

- Any breast lump or thickening that feels different from the surrounding tissue
- A change in the shape or size of a breast
- Puckering or dimpling of breast skin
- If the nipple turns inward into the breast – inverted nipple
- Peeling, scaling or flaking of the nipple or breast skin
- Discharge or fluid from the nipple - especially if it's bloody
- Redness or pitting of the skin over the breast like the skin of an orange.

## BREAST SELF-EXAMINATION (BSE)

Breast Self-Examination should be practiced once a month. If you menstruate, do it two or three days after the end of your period, when your breasts are least likely to be tender or swollen. If you are not menstruating, due to: menopause, surgical menopause, amenorrhea, or other cause, choose a day such as the first of the month, and perform breast self-examination each month on that day.

## VISUAL

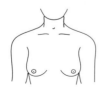

**1.** Stand before the mirror. Inspect both breasts for anything unusual, such as discharge from the nipples, rash or puckering, dimpling, or scaling of the skin.

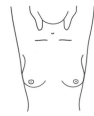

**2.** Watching closely in the mirror, raise both arms over your head, stretching them up high. Examine both breasts and the underarm area.

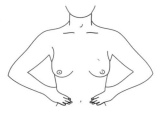

**3.** Next press hands firmly on the hips and bow slightly toward the mirror as you pull your shoulders and elbows forward.

## PALPATION

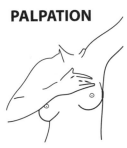

**4.** Raise your left arm. Use three or four fingers of your right hand to explore your left breast firmly, carefully and thoroughly feeling for any unusual lump or mass under the skin. Beginning at the outer edge, press the flat part of your fingers in small circles, moving the circles slowly around the breast. Pay attention to the tail of the breast (the area between the breast and armpit) and the armpit. Repeat this for the right breast using your left hand.

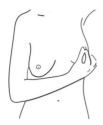

**5.** Gently squeeze the nipple of your left breast and look for a discharge. Repeat this for your right breast. You should see your health care practitioner if you have any discharge during the month.

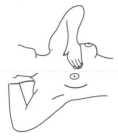

**6.** Repeat steps 4 and 5 lying flat on your back with your arm over your head and a pillow or folded towel under the shoulder of the breast that you are examining. This position flattens the breast tissue making it easier to examine. Use the same circular motion described above in step 4. Do this for left and right breast.

If you find anything suspicious, or have any questions, report it to your health care practitioner immediately.

## CAUSES

### Reduce your Exposure to Environmental Estrogen

Thank goodness the newscasts and newspapers are finally reporting about the estrogen-mimicking or xenoestrogenic (pronounced "zeeno-estrogenic") effects of certain chemicals. I'm sure you are aware of the concern about bisphenol-A found in plastic baby bottles, water bottles and the lining of canned foods. Research continues to link this chemical to dangerous health consequences. A 2010 report handily demonstrated that bisphenol-A encourages abnormal proliferation in human breast epithelial cells.

Other chemicals to avoid include phthalates (pronounced "thay-lates") which are frequently used in hairspray, deodorant, nail polish and cologne formulations. They can be inhaled or absorbed through the skin and are known to damage the liver, lungs and reproductive organs. In little boys, phthalates have been linked to undescended testes, which must be surgically corrected. Phthalates have also been shown to affect the quantity and quality of sperm. Be watchful of the word 'fragrance' on the labels of body care and home care products. This word typically replaces up to 200 chemical ingredients, and phthalates are often in the mix.

Avoid these xenoestrogens!

- Phthalates: monobutyl phthalate, monobenzyl phthalate, monoethyl phthalate and diethyl phthalate
- Parabens: butylparaben, ethylparaben, methylparaben, propylparaben, isopropylparaben and isobutylparaben
- Sunscreen chemicals: benzophenone-3 (Bp-3), homosalate (HMS), 4-methyl-benzylidene camphor (4-MBC), octyl-methoxycinnamate (OMC), and octyl-dimethyl-PABA (OD-PABA). Animals exposed to these chemicals experienced an increased proliferation of MCF-7 breast cancer cells.

The paraben family of chemicals are used extensively in body and beauty care products because they are cheap and plentiful – and typically don't cause a skin reaction. Used as preservatives and plasticizers, these chemicals are considered safe, yet they are proven to exert estrogenic activity on females and males alike. All six parabens listed above stimulate the growth of breast-cancer causing MCF-7 cells. As well, parabens have been found intact in human breast cells. Studies also show that parabens cause a drop in testosterone levels in men and damage the final stages of sperm production.

Mineral oil is another ingredient to avoid, because, as a petrochemical product, it may contain xenoestrogenic polycyclic aromatic hydrocarbons (PAH). These are the same chemicals found in charbroiled meats. PAHs are also used to make dyes, medicines, pesticides and plastics. Some PAHs are known to activate estrogen receptors. A 2004 study found that PAHs stimulated the proliferation of MCF-7 breast cancer cells.

While you are making your shopping list to replace xenoestrogen products in your cupboards, be sure to write down unbleached paper products like toilet paper, feminine pads, tampons and tissues to reduce your exposure to dioxins. Chlorinated dioxins are a by-product of bleaching of pulp and paper and are linked to disruption of the hormonal system, birth defects and miscarriage. Several studies have highlighted a connection between dioxins and endometriosis and they've been associated with an increase in cancer-causing metabolites in breast cancer cells.

Although many xenoestrogens are used at levels that cause no observable effect (NOE), studies show that combining xenoestrogens in the various products you would use throughout the day has an additive effect. In fact, research indicates that combining a variety of xenoestrogens below NOE produces an estrogen-mimic effect. Learn to read labels and avoid products containing these chemicals.

## 💡 FACT – Did You Know?

A study published in the *Journal of the National Cancer Institute* June 2000 found that women with advanced breast cancer, had increased levels of the stress hormone cortisol. They had a significantly earlier death than patients with normal levels. The researchers also found that the women with increased cortisol levels had few Natural Killer (NK) cells and the immune system was less able to fight the cancer cells. In other words, REDUCE YOUR STRESS!

## TESTS and DIAGNOSIS

While the safety of mammograms continues to be assessed, other imaging tests to consider include an ultrasound, thermography or MRI for early screening. Remember to perform breast self exams once a month. Over 80% of most breast problems are found through self-examination.

### *Mammography*

A mammogram is an x-ray of the breast and is commonly used to screen for breast cancer. It typically picks up lesions as small as 0.5 cm, which are usually not palpable through a breast exam. Mammograms can detect approximately 85% of all breast cancers whereas an experienced physician can detect 61 to 92% of breast cancers through a routine breast exam. However, some women are choosing other screening tools for several reasons. One reason is that mammograms may be less accurate in picking up lesions in smaller breasts and can miss up to 25% of tumours in women 40 to 49 years of age. False negative results may occur as well. One study found that women who had a mammogram during the last two weeks of the menstrual cycle were twice as likely to have false negative results – meaning that the x-ray was interpreted to be fine but cancer was actually present and the tumours missed. The other dilemma is that mammograms do require small doses of radiation, which can accumulate over time and increase the risk of developing breast cancer. It may take 40 years for cancer to show up after exposure to radiation, so for women under the age of 50 receiving annual mammograms, this may pose a risk.

### *Breast Ultrasound*

An ultrasound uses sound waves to produce images of structures deep within the body and can help determine whether a breast abnormality is likely to be a fluid-filled cyst (typically non-cancerous) or a solid mass (may be cancerous). Ultrasounds are ideal at examining a lump or area of concern that has already been identified by a physical exam or mammography but are not so useful as a whole breast-screening tool. They are generally safe and there is no radiation exposure. If the ultrasound finds a lump that is filled with fluid, a biopsy is not necessary. However, if it shows that the mass is solid, then a biopsy is conducted to determine whether the lump is a fibroadenoma or cancer. An ultrasound may be used before a mammogram when a cyst is suspected and therefore, a patient can be spared exposure to radiation.

## *MRI*

An MRI uses magnet and radio waves to create pictures of the interior of your breast. MRIs are more useful and accurate in women in their 20s and 30s who may have denser breasts and a higher genetic susceptibility. MRIs do not use radiation but instead use a huge magnet to image tissues after a contrast dye is injected intravenously. The dye is typically absorbed more easily by cancer cells than by normal or benign tissues. Some disadvantages to the breast MRI are that they are expensive, they produce a high level of false positive results and there is much interpretation needed by doctors and technicians.

## *Breast Thermography*

Breast Thermography, also known as Medical Digital Infrared Thermal Imaging, is a noninvasive diagnostic technique that allows the examiner to visualize and quantify changes in skin surface temperature. A specialized digital infrared camera is used and provides a detailed 'picture' of the heat levels and patterns of the breast tissue. It is non-invasive, no radiation is emitted to the patient and there is no contact to the breasts in contrast to the mammogram. By using the digital infrared imaging scans, the function, physiology and metabolism of the breast tissue can be assessed.

Abnormal cells are usually hotter than normal cells. This is because malignant tissue needs more blood supply and new blood vessels grow to feed this increased demand. This is called angiogenesis ("angio" meaning blood vessel and "genesis" meaning creation). Thermography will show the difference between normal breast tissue and problem areas.

Thermography fills a gap in clinical diagnosis. While x-rays, CT scans, ultrasound and MRI are tests of anatomy, thermography is unique in its capability to show physiological change and metabolic processes. It has also proven to be a very useful complementary procedure to other diagnostic modalities.

Canadian studies done at the Ville Marie Breast Center in Montreal have found that thermography was positive for 83% of breast cancers, compared to 61% for clinical breast exams alone and 84% for mammograms. When thermography was used in combination with a mammogram, the detection rate was increased to 95%.

### Biopsy

A biopsy will confirm the presence of cancer if the above tests have not been definitive. During a biopsy, a tissue sample of the suspicious breast cells is taken and sent for lab testing to determine whether the cells are cancerous. Sometimes a lumpectomy is performed if the breast mass has been identified early and it has been confirmed that the cancer has not spread. The whole mass is then removed, with a large enough margin of normal tissue to be certain that all the cancer cells have been included.

### PREVENTION and TREATMENT – Dietary and Lifestyle

## FOOD FACTORS

Perhaps the most exciting new research on nutrition to reduce cancer risk involves carbohydrate consumption. Researchers have set out to determine whether a diet high in carbohydrates, resulting in chronically elevated insulin, would affect breast cancer risk by stimulating insulin receptors or through insulin-like growth factor. In several studies throughout the world, involving almost 150,000 women, scientists concluded that there is indeed an association between high Glycemic Index (GI) foods (see **Appendix**) and breast cancer. This was especially evident among premenopausal women (under age 50) who were overweight (BMI greater than 25) or had a large waist circumference. Since a low GI diet is a healthy diet with plenty of options for fruits, vegetables, whole grains and lean sources of protein, it's an easy switch to make to promote your health.

Highly refined sugars such as white flour, soft drinks, canned juices, candy, chocolate bars, donuts and cookies can have a huge impact on immune function, especially on the body's white blood cells (the body's defense mechanism). The number of phagocytes (a special type of white blood cell) decreases within 30 minutes after ingestion of sweets and can last for over five hours. A reduction in white blood cells can lead to a poorly functioning immune system and leave the body highly vulnerable to infection and disease.

A large class of chemicals found in fruits and vegetables (phytochemicals) have been shown to be beneficial in the prevention and treatment of breast cancer. The brassica family contains vegetables such as broccoli, cauliflower, Brussels sprouts, bok choy, kale, watercress, radish, kohlrabi and collards. All have very potent healing properties. A chemical called indole-3-carbinol is found in the above vegetables and helps to inactivate potential harmful estrogens preventing breast cancer. Sulforaphane, found in broccoli and broccoli sprouts, Brussels sprouts and cauliflower, increases the ability of the liver's detoxifying enzymes to remove toxin substances from the body. For those with an underactive thyroid or goiter, caution is advised when consuming raw brassicas, although they are fine when lightly cooked. In some people, they may interfere with thyroid function. Ingesting sea vegetables and other sources of iodine can prevent this complication.

Garlic has been proven to inhibit the growth of both estrogen positive and estrogen receptor (ER)-negative breast cancer cells. Garlic is high in the trace minerals selenium and germanium, both of which help reduce the risk of cancer. It contains protective antioxidants, isoflavones and allyl sulfides. Garlic, onions and leeks contain compounds which help the liver in its detoxification pathways.

Lycopene is a potent antioxidant and gives the red colour to fruits and vegetables in which it is present. These include tomatoes, watermelon, pink grapefruit, guava and rosehip. Tomatoes are the highest source of lycopene but it is more bioavailable when the tomatoes are heated and processed into sauces. Research has shown lycopene protects against cancer (breast, cervix, mouth, pharynx, esophagus, stomach, bladder, colon, rectum) by stopping cell division in cancer cells.

Fibre is found in fruits, vegetables, legumes, grains, nuts and seeds and is important in the prevention of breast cancer as well as many other conditions (see **Appendix**). Sufficient fibre in the diet reduces the amount of circulating estrogen in the blood by binding and eliminating it through the bowels. Diets high in fibre and complex carbohydrates stabilize blood sugar and improve insulin sensitivity, which will improve estrogen dominance. Fibre improves "good bacteria" in the bowel thus reducing reabsorption of estrogen in the body.

Many herbs and spices are very beneficial in the prevention of cancer especially breast cancer. Turmeric has been used in East Indian cooking, traditional Chinese medicine as well as Ayurvedic medicine. It has antioxidant, antitumor and anti-inflammatory properties. Turmeric protects the liver and improves liver detoxification. Rosemary increases the 2-hydroxylation of estradiol and estrone to form more of the "good" C-2 estrogens and decrease the formation of "bad" C-16 estrogens. Sage is a powerful immune tonic. Ginger helps with digestion, is anti-inflammatory, an immune stimulant, and aids in detoxification in the liver.

New research underlines the crucial role of Vitamin D in promoting breast health. Studies show that Vitamin D not only kills breast cancer cells, it also inhibits metastasis and tumour angiogenesis, the mechanism a cancer tumour uses to feed itself. Vitamin D decreases the stimulatory effect of 17beta-estradiol and inhibits MCF-7 cancer cell growth. Research also shows that Vitamin D reduces the 17beta-estradiol-mediated increase in breast cancer susceptibility gene (BRCA1) protein. Finally, research done on women aged 18 to 22 years, found that higher levels of vitamin D may reduce progesterone and estradiol, providing a potential means of reducing breast cancer in young women.

And while you haven't heard a lot about vitamin $K_3$ yet, get ready! Health benefits of this mysterious vitamin are gaining attention as research unravels its importance. Studies show that $K_3$ not only induces cancer cell death but, along with vitamin D, slows down growth of MCF-7 breast cancer cells while boosting activity of antioxidant enzymes.

### *Phytoestrogens*

Phytoestrogens are plant versions of the human hormone estrogen. They're considered to be weak estrogenic compounds with an average of about 2% of the strength of estrogens. They can be beneficial when estrogen levels are either too high or too low. When metabolized, they bind on the same cellular sites as do estrogens, altering estrogenic effects. The three main classes of phytoestrogens are isoflavones, lignans and coumestans. Isoflavones are the most widely studied class of phytoestrogens, with genistein and daidzein providing most of the data. The best food sources of phytoestrogens are non-genetically engineered organic soybeans, flax seeds, oats, rye, lentils, fennel, chickpeas, alfalfa and sesame.

There has been much controversy recently about soy and concerns about its safety. These concerns are based on its weak estrogenic and hormonal effects. Several studies have concluded that Asian women who consume a traditional low-fat, high-soy diet have a four- to six- fold lower risk of developing breast cancer. The dietary phytoestrogens have also been shown to inhibit cancer growth by competing with estradiol for the type II estrogen binding sites.

Recent data from the Women's Healthy Eating and Living (WHEL) Study were used to examine the effect of soy intake on breast cancer prognosis in 3,088 breast cancer survivors. These women were early stage breast cancer patients who were followed for an average of 7.3 years. The association between soy intake and breast cancer recurrence and/or death was then tracked. The study found that as soy isoflavone intake increased, the risk of death decreased. Women at the highest levels of soy had a 54% reduction in risk of death.

The type and frequency of soy consumed is important. My recommendation to patients is to choose organic, non-GMO forms of soy as well as fermented soy products such as tempeh or miso. I also recommend eating soy in moderation, meaning between 50 to 150 mg of isoflavones (phytoestrogens) daily. For example, one cup of regular soymilk contains 30 mg and half a cup of tofu will contain 35 mg of isoflavones. Before making any conclusions about soy, it's important to remember that every woman is different and what may work for one woman may not for the other. Some women may have soy allergies and for this reason, may not be able to tolerate it due to difficulty with digestion.

## LIFESTYLE TIPS

- Reduce weight if you are overweight or obese. Stick to a low GI diet. Follow the low GI foods (see **Appendix** – *Low Glycemic Index Food Chart*).

- Minimize alcohol consumption.

- Quit smoking.

- Exercise at least 40 to 60 minutes per day, at least three times weekly. Practice yoga or Qigong to improve energy flow, lymphatics and healing. Combine with aerobic and weight-bearing exercises.

- Choose bras that do not have an underwire or choose one that is loose fitting. Reduce bra-wearing time by taking the bra off as soon as you are home from work.

- Use castor oil packs over the liver and breasts three or more times a week to improve lymphatic circulation and reduce cysts (see **Appendix**).

- Do a cleanse at least once a year to detoxify heavy metals and other chemicals from the bowels, kidneys and liver.

- Reduce your exposure to xenoestrogenic petrochemicals used in pesticides, herbicides and fertilizers by choosing organic foods.

- Decrease your exposure to dioxins by avoiding bleached varieties of toiletries and feminine products. Choose body and home care products without xenoestrogenic chemicals. Do not buy clothes that need to be dry-cleaned.

- Use home and body care products that are not xenoestrogenic. Visit the Environmental Working Group website *www.ewg.com* or *www. environmentaldefence.ca* for more information about safe products.

- Relax with a soothing herbal tea made with hibiscus flowers, shepherd's purse, raspberry leaves, vitex berries, orange peels and yarrow herbs and flowers to help balance hormones.

- Avoid synthetic hormone replacement therapy that involves the use of estrogen and progestin. Use herbal alternatives for menopausal symptoms. (see **Menopause** Chapter)

- Avoid using the birth control pill to prevent contraception or to treat acne. Investigate other forms of contraception (see **Birth Control** Chapter).

- Make sure your diet contains adequate fibre, as this will help you eliminate excess estrogen.

- Grind two tablespoons of flaxseed daily and add it to your cereal, yogurt or salad. Flax is an excellent source of lignan precursors which can help prevent the development of breast cancer and other cancers.

## KEY SUPPLEMENTS

### Calcium-D-glucarate

Calcium-D-glucarate is the calcium salt of D-glucaric acid produced naturally in small amounts by humans. It is found in many fruits and vegetables, with the highest concentrations in oranges, apples, grapefruit and cruciferous vegetables. Research has shown that this compound inhibits beta-glucuronidase, an enzyme produced by the flora in the colon

*Mind/Body Connection*

Breast issues often relate to over-mothering or over-protecting others. Allow others the freedom to be who they are.

and involved in Phase II of liver detoxification. A high level of the enzyme beta-glucuronidase is associated with a higher risk of hormone-dependent cancers such as breast, prostate and colon cancer. Calcium-D-glucarate is also involved in estrogen metabolism and has lipid-lowering properties.

DOSAGE: *450–1500 mg daily*

### Indole-3-carbinol

Indole-3-carbinol (I3C) is a compound found in vegetables of the Brassaca family including broccoli, cauliflower, Brussels sprouts, cabbage and kale. I3C supports liver detoxification and healthy estrogen metabolism by increasing the ratio of 2-hydroxy estrogens ("good" estrogens) to 16-hydroxy estrogens ("bad" estrogens).

DOSAGE: *200–500 mg daily*

### Green Tea Extract

Green tea contains polyphenols and epigallocatechin-3-gallate, which have been found to regulate cancer cell replication and induce apoptosis (programmed cell death).

DOSAGE: *300–700 mg daily*

### Turmeric – *Curcuma longa*

Turmeric has a long tradition of use in the Chinese and Ayurvedic systems of medicine, particularly as an anti-inflammatory agent, and for the treatment of flatulence, jaundice, menstrual difficulties, hematuria, hemorrhage and colic. Turmeric can also be applied topically in poultices to relieve pain and inflammation. Current research has focussed on turmeric's antioxidant, hepato-protective, anti-inflammatory, anticarcinogenic, and antimicrobial properties, in addition to its use in cardiovascular disease and gastrointestinal disorders.

DOSAGE: *up to 1500 mg daily*

## Milk Thistle – *Silybum marianum*

Milk thistle is one of the most well-known liver protective herbs and has been shown to benefit digestion, the spleen and the kidneys. Flavonoids present in milk thistle, bind to liver cells and protect them from being injured by foreign chemicals thus preventing cirrhosis and inflammation. Milk thistle contains silymarin, which is composed of the flavanolignans silybin, silydianin, and silychristine, with silybin being the most biologically active. Silymarin is found in highest concentrations in the fruit portion of the plant but is also found in the leaves and seeds. In laboratory studies, silymarin has been found to stabilize cell membranes, thus preventing toxic chemicals from entering the cell. Laboratory studies have demonstrated that silymarin stimulates synthesis and activity of enzymes responsible for detoxification pathways and exhibits antioxidant properties. Silymarin has also been shown to neutralize a wide range of free radicals.

Laboratory experiments conducted using cancer cell lines have suggested that silybin enhances the efficacy of the chemotherapy drugs cisplatin and doxorubicin against ovarian and breast cancer cells. Silybin appears to have direct anticancer effects against prostate, breast and ectocervical tumour cells. Silybin may also affect the cell cycle in cancer cells by slowing down cell growth, as demonstrated with prostate cancer cell lines.

DOSAGE: *400–600 mg daily*

## Rosemary Extract

Rosemary increases the 2-hydroxy estrogens ("good") and decreases the 16-hydroxy estrogens ("bad"). It also supports phase II detoxification improving estrogen elimination and metabolism.

DOSAGE: *up to 100 mg daily*

## DIM

DIM is naturally occurring in cruciferous vegetables such as broccoli. It has been shown to increase the production of "good" estrogens and decrease "bad" estrogens. DIM has powerful anti-cancer effects in both breast and cervical cancer.

DOSAGE: *up to 300 mg daily*

## Lycopene

Lycopene is a potent antioxidant and gives the red colour to fruits and vegetables. These include tomatoes, watermelon, pink grapefruit, guava and rosehip. Tomatoes are the highest source of lycopene. It is more bioavailable when the tomatoes are heated and processed into sauces. Research has shown lycopene protects against cancer (breast, cervix, mouth, pharynx, esophagus, stomach, bladder, colon, rectum) by stopping cell division in cancer cells. One study found that by consuming 6.5 mg of lycopene daily, breast cancer was reduced by 36%. Tomatoes are part of the nightshade family and may aggravate inflammatory conditions such as arthritis.

DOSAGE: *up to 15 mg daily*

## Sulforaphane

Sulforaphane is another compound that is naturally found in the brassica family of vegetables. It contains isothiocyanates, which are sulfur-containing phytochemicals that prevent DNA damage and block the growth of tumours initiated by environmental toxins. Sulforaphane is a natural antioxidant and induces phase II detoxification in the liver, which helps to eliminate harmful toxins from the body. Some research has shown that sulforaphane can actually initiate apoptosis, programmed cell death on cancer cells and prevent further cancer growth.

DOSAGE: *600 mcg daily*

****All the above nutrients are found in* **EstroSense®**, *an excellent product for supporting healthy liver detoxification, estrogen metabolism and preventing estrogen dominant conditions.*

## Chaste Tree Berry - *Vitex agnus castus*

Chaste Tree Berry (*Vitex*) has an effect on the hypothalamus/hypophysis axis in which it increases luteinizing hormone and progesterone. By increasing progesterone levels, excess estrogen decreases and this may prevent and reduce the risk of developing estrogen-dependent conditions such as breast cancer.

DOSAGE: *Take up to 400 mg daily.*

## Modified Citrus Pectin - MCP

Modified citrus pectin, also known as fractionated pectin, is a compound obtained from the peel and pulp of citrus fruits. Research indicates that in order for cancer to grow, divide and migrate (metastasize), cancer cells must first clump together (aggregate) with helper cells called galectins. MCP is thought to have an affinity for galectins on the surface of the cancer cells and thus block cancer cell aggregation, growth and metastasis. This effect has been shown in certain cancers such as melanomas, prostate and breast cancers.

DOSAGE: *at least 15 grams daily in three divided doses*

## Vitamin D3

A recent study on vitamin D and breast cancer risk was published in the *American Journal of Clinical Nutrition 2010* that once again points the way to vitamin D as a safe and important strategy in lowering breast cancer risk. The study included about 6,500 women between the ages of 25 and 74. Approximately half the women were diagnosed with breast cancer and half were not. According to the study results, a vitamin D supplement intake greater than 400 IU/day compared with no vitamin D supplement intake reduced the risk of breast cancer by about 25%. This Canadian population-based, case-control study also observed that calcium supplementation did not influence breast cancer risk.

DOSAGE: *2000 IU daily*

## Coenzyme Q10 - Ubiquinone

Coenzyme Q10 (ubiquinone, CoQ10) is an important antioxidant necessary for the health of all human tissues and organs. It is required for the production of ATP, our body's energy source.

Research has shown that women with low levels of CoQ10 have a corresponding poor prognosis. In this study, 200 women with breast tumours (80 malignant and 120 benign) found that CoQ10 concentrations were reduced both in patients with cancer and in women with benign lesions, compared to the control population of women with normal tissue.

DOSAGE: *300 mg daily*

## Alpha Lipoic Acid

Alpha lipoic acid (ALA) is a potent antioxidant that has the ability to increase the effectiveness and lifespan of many other antioxidants including vitamins C and E, quercetin and CoQ10. It also promotes the production of glutathione, another powerful antioxidant and liver detoxifier. ALA is an important immune booster as it increases the number of T helper cells, which help protect our body from environmental insult. ALA can reduce the toxic side effects of chemotherapy, help to regenerate the liver and can bind to many heavy metals and remove them from the body. These metals include lead, aluminum, mercury, copper, cadmium and arsenic.

DOSAGE: *300 mg daily*

## Melatonin - *SleepSense®*

Melatonin appears to increase the survival time and improve quality of life in patients with various types of cancer, including non-small cell lung cancer, gastric cancer, hepatocellular carcinoma, metastatic breast cancer, melanoma and brain metastases due to solid tumours.

Some believe that melatonin competes with estrogen for the estrogen receptors thus preventing excess estrogen activity in the body. When used in combination with tamoxifen, melatonin has been shown to increase the effectiveness of the drug and improve the response to chemotherapy.

DOSAGE: *3–20 mg taken before bed.*

## Flaxseed Oil and/or Pure Fish Oil

Essential fatty acids in the form of flaxseed or uncontaminated fish oil decrease the formation of PGE2, a type of prostaglandin that acts as a messenger molecule to promote inflammatory pathways in the body. Prostaglandins are made by every one of our cells and can either feed pathways that create disease or restore health. Some prostaglandins can actually inhibit cancer growth and support healthy immune function, while others promote cancer. Omega-3s found in fish and flax oil support the "healthy" prostaglandin pathways, preventing disease and abnormal cell growth.

DOSAGE: *Take up to 2 Tbsp of flax oil daily and/or up to 3000 mg fish oil daily with a minimum of 1000 mg EPA and 600 mg DHA.*

## Probiotics - *Lactobacillus acidophilus* and *Bifidobacterium* spp.

Probiotics are known to have an important role in the maintenance of normal flora in the gastrointestinal tract. Along with adequate dietary fibre, they are involved in the detoxification of excess estrogens from the body via the bowel. This may be beneficial in preventing estrogen-dominant conditions. Probiotics also support optimal immune function as 70% of our immune cells do reside in our gut!

DOSAGE: *at least 10 billion CFU daily with food*

## Vitamin C

Vitamin C has been well researched for its potent antioxidant role for the treatment of many cancers. It helps to enhance immune function and exerts protection against environmental carcinogens and has anti-viral effects. Vitamin C can protect against cancers by preventing tumour growth and the formation of metastases by building connective tissue. This vitamin increases the activity of white blood cells thus improving overall immunity.

DOSAGE: *up to 6000 mg daily or to bowel tolerance.*

## Vitamin K

Both *in vitro* and *in vivo* studies have shown that vitamin K exhibits anticancer effects. A number of cancer cell lines (liver, colon, leukemia, lung, stomach, lymphocyte, nasopharynx, breast and oral epidermoid) have been investigated for inhibition by vitamin K.

DOSAGE: *up to 300 mcg daily*

## Selenium

Numerous populations around the globe have developed selenium deficiencies due to the fact that many areas now have soil that is deficient in this trace mineral. Deficiencies in selenium have been associated with a higher incidence in many cancers. This mineral has an important role in repairing DNA damage and increasing the immune response protecting the body from environmental substances.

DOSAGE: *200 mcg twice daily*

## B Vitamins – B Complex

The B vitamins are needed to convert carbohydrates into glucose, giving the body energy. They also support immune function. Since the birth control pill depletes the body of B vitamins, many women who are taking the pill have lower amounts of these important vitamins. This can have adverse effects on estrogen metabolism as the B vitamins are needed for liver detoxification pathways and the breakdown of excess estrogen into less harmful forms.

DOSAGE: *50 mg of a B complex two to three times daily*

## Adrenal Support – *AdrenaSense*®

Supporting adrenal function will help to normalize the stress hormone cortisol thus preventing cancers that may be due to stress, such as breast cancer. Since Natural Killer cells are sensitive to increased cortisol levels, a strong immune system is linked to healthy adrenal function.

DOSAGE: *Take 1-3 capsules daily with food.*

## CONVENTIONAL MEDICINE

### Breast Cancer Surgery

- A lumpectomy may be performed to remove the tumour. The surgeon includes a small margin of surrounding healthy tissue to be certain that all the cancer cells are removed. A lumpectomy is usually reserved for smaller tumours that are easily separated from the surrounding tissue.
- A mastectomy removes the entire breast including the lobules, ducts, fatty tissue and some skin, along with the nipple and areola. If the cancer is more advanced, a radical mastectomy is performed in which the underlying muscle of the chest wall is removed along with the breast tissue and surrounding lymph nodes. Some women will choose to have both breasts removed to prevent recurrence in either breast.

### Chemotherapy

- Chemotherapy uses drugs to destroy cancer cells. If the cancer has a high chance of returning or spreading to another area of the body, this therapy may be suggested to reduce the possibility that the cancer will recur. Chemotherapy is usually recommended after surgery but is sometimes started beforehand with women who have large breast tumours. The goal is to shrink the tumour to a size that will make it easier to remove with surgery.

## Radiation

- Radiation uses high-powered beams of energy to kill cancer cells and is usually recommended after chemotherapy to destroy any cancer cells near the original site.

## Drugs

- Medications can be used after surgery or other treatments to decrease the chance of the cancer returning.
- Tamoxifen is the most commonly used selective estrogen receptor modulator (SERM). SERMs act by blocking estrogen from attaching to the estrogen receptor on the cancer cells, slowing the growth of tumours and killing tumour cells. Possible side effects include fatigue, hot flashes, night sweats and vaginal dryness.
- Aromatase inhibitors block the enzyme that converts androgens in the body into estrogen after menopause. The following drugs are effective only in postmenopausal women: anastrozole (Arimidex), letrozole (Femara) and exemestane (Aromasin). Side effects include joint and muscle pain, as well as an increased risk of osteoporosis.
- Trastuzumab (Herceptin) targets a protein called human growth factor receptor 2 (HER2). HER2 helps breast cancer cells grow and survive. Side effects may include heart damage, headaches and skin rashes.
- Goserelin can cause artificial menopause by lowering the pituitary gland's production of LH and FSH that stimulate the ovaries to produce estrogen and progesterone.

# CHAPTER 5

# CERVICAL DYSPLASIA

Cervical dysplasia refers to pre-cancerous changes in the cells on the surface of the cervix that are seen under a microscope. The cervix is the lower part of the uterus that opens at the top of the vagina. A Pap test, performed by a medical professional during an annual physical exam, can detect these abnormal cellular changes.

Cervical dysplasia can progress to cervical cancer, a common cancer that is the second most common cancer in women ages 20 to 39 if left untreated. Cervical cancer is one of the most common causes of cancer deaths among women, particularly in impoverished countries such as India and Brazil. Internationally, invasive cervical cancer accounts for 11.6% of all cancers. Almost all cases of cervical dysplasia are caused by the human papilloma virus (HPV) but not all women with the virus will develop cervical dysplasia or cervical cancer.

The following may increase your risk of cervical dysplasia and cancer:

- Becoming sexually active before age 18
- Having multiple sexual partners or being sexually active with a man who has multiple sexual partners
- Giving birth before age 22
- Smoking
- Compromised immune system

- Low socio-economic status
- Family history of cervical cancer
- Oral contraceptives
- Obesity
- Poor nutrition
- Chlamydia infection, herpes simplex virus or HIV.

### FACT – Did You Know?

Women who smoke are about twice as likely to develop cervical cancer. Smoking also depletes vitamin C, an important antioxidant for cancer prevention.

## SIGNS and SYMPTOMS

Women typically do not experience any signs or symptoms of cervical dysplasia and early cervical cancer generally does not produce any symptoms. As cancer progresses though, the following signs and symptoms of more advanced cervical cancer may appear:

- Vaginal bleeding after intercourse, between periods or after menopause
- Watery, bloody vaginal discharge that may be heavy or have a foul odour
- Pelvic pain or pain during intercourse.

It is always important to schedule an appointment with a medical professional if you have any signs or symptoms that are worrisome.

## CAUSES

Almost 100% of cervical dysplasias and cancers are caused by HPV. There are currently over 100 HPV subtypes that have been identified and categorized in which over 30 can infect the genital area. The low-risk types are generally associated with external genital warts but do not cause cervical cancer.

## TESTS and DIAGNOSIS

A Pap test during a routine annual physical exam will screen for cervical dysplasia or cancer. Pap smears should be performed approximately three years after the onset of vaginal intercourse and no later than 21 years of age. During a Pap test, the doctor brushes cells from the cervix and sends the sample to the lab to be examined for abnormalities. The test can detect abnormal cells in the cervix, including cancer cells that can increase the risk of cervical cancer.

If abnormal cells are detected, the doctor may use another test called the HPV DNA test to determine whether you are infected with any of the types of HPV that are most likely to lead to cervical cancer.

Cervical dysplasia that is seen on a Pap smear is called squamous intraepithelial lesion (SIL) and may be graded as:

- Low-grade (LSIL)
- High-grade (HSIL)
- Possibly cancerous (malignant).

If a Pap smear shows abnormal cells or cervical dysplasia, further testing is usually recommended:

- Follow-up Pap smears - every three to six months may be recommended for mild cases.
- Colposcopy-directed biopsy – the removal of a sample of unusual cells from the cervix using special biopsy tools to confirm diagnosis.
- Cone biopsy may be performed after colposcopy - involves taking a cone-shaped sample of the cervix to obtain deeper layers of the cervical cells for lab testing.

Dysplasia that is confirmed from a biopsy of the cervix is called cervical intraepithelial neoplasia (CIN) and is grouped into 3 categories:

- CIN I – mild dysplasia
- CIN II – moderate dysplasia

- CIN III – severe dysplasia to carcinoma *in situ*.

*Note: Low-grade lesions (CIN I) usually regress but may still progress to cervical cancer. High-grade lesions (CIN II or III) are more likely to progress to cervical cancer.

If cervical cancer is confirmed, further testing is suggested to determine whether the cancer has spread and to what extent – this process is called staging. Stages of cervical cancer include:

- Stage I – Cancer is confined to the cervix.
- Stage II – Cancer includes the cervix and uterus, but has not spread to the pelvic wall or the lower portion of the vagina.
- Stage III – Cancer at this stage has moved beyond the cervix and uterus to the pelvic wall or the lower portion of the vagina.
- Stage IV – At this stage, cancer has spread to nearby organs, such as the bladder or rectum, or it has spread to other areas of the body, such as the lungs, liver or bones.

## Screening Guidelines

- Screening should begin at age 21 or approximately three years after first sexual contact.
- Pap tests should be performed once a year until three normal results have occurred consecutively, then every two years.
- If a woman has not been screened in more than five years, she should be screened annually until there are three consecutive negative Pap tests.
- Women with previous abnormal Pap tests may be screened more frequently – every six months.
- Screening may be discontinued after the age of 70 if there has been an adequate negative screening history in the previous 10 years.
- Even if a woman is not sexually active, she should continue to have Pap tests.

## PREVENTION and TREATMENT – Dietary and Lifestyle

### FOOD FACTORS

A diet high in fruits and vegetables has been found to be protective against cervical cancer and dysplasia. Foods high in vitamin C, selenium, carotenoids and vitamin E should be included as part of every woman's diet.

- Vitamin C: papaya, kiwi, peppers, oranges, broccoli, Brussels sprouts, grapefruit, strawberries and cantaloupe
- Selenium: Brazil nuts, fish, turkey, barley, shrimp, lamb and scallops
- Vitamin E: Sunflower seeds, almonds, spinach, Swiss chard, turnip greens, papaya, mustard greens, avocado, collard greens and asparagus
- Carotenoids: carrots, squash, collards, tomatoes, sweet potato, pumpkin, spinach and kale

Indole-3-carbinol/DIM found in cruciferous vegetables such as broccoli, cabbage, Brussels sprouts, cauliflower and kale is protective against many female cancers. Including these foods in the diet helps support healthy estrogen metabolism and conversion of harmful estrogen metabolites into safer ones. Women with CIN I or II typically have altered estrogen metabolism and have higher amounts of 16alpha-hydroxyestrone (a carcinogen) and less 2-hydroxyestrone (protective).

A folic acid deficiency has been associated with a higher risk of cervical dysplasia. Women who are taking oral contraceptives are usually low in folic acid amongst other vitamins and minerals because they are depleted. Include foods high in folic acid such as: brewer's yeast, black-eyed peas, lentils, lima beans, kidney beans, dandelion greens and leeks.

EGCG is a polyphenol present in green tea. Smaller studies confirm regression of cervical lesions. Choose green tea over caffeinated beverages such as coffee or tea.

### LIFESTYLE TIPS

- Have routine Pap tests – at least every one to two years for a normal

Pap and every three to six months for an abnormal Pap. After three consecutive Pap tests, resume to one to two years.

- Quit smoking.
- Minimize alcohol consumption.
- Consider other forms of birth control if taking oral contraceptives. Use barrier methods, such as male or female condoms to decrease exposure to HPV.
- Support healthy liver function – cleanse one to two times per year.
- Reduce stress and practice stress management techniques such as deep breathing exercises, yoga or meditation.
- Exercise at least 40 to 60 minutes per day (three times a week minimum) with a combination of cardio and weight-bearing exercises.

## KEY SUPPLEMENTS

### Folic Acid

Studies have shown a connection between a folic acid deficiency and an increased risk of cervical dysplasia. In two double-blind trials and one uncontrolled trial, folic acid in doses of 5-10 mg/day for one to three months, was found to be an effective treatment for CIN in women taking oral contraceptives. Deficiencies in folic acid are seen more commonly in women who are taking oral contraceptives and therefore, those women should definitely supplement with folic acid. Folic acid along with vitamin B12 and B6 decrease high levels of homocysteine, which has also been associated with an increased risk of cervical cancer.

DOSAGE: *2-10 mg daily for treatment or 1-3 mg for prevention*

### Vitamin C

Vitamin C exerts both anticancer and antiviral effects. As well, it is involved in collagen synthesis and helps to detoxify potential carcinogens. Therefore, Vitamin C has the potential to be beneficial for women with cervical dysplasia.

DOSAGE: *2000–5000 mg daily or to bowel tolerance*

## Carotenes

Studies of cervical dysplasia and carotenoids indicate low concentrations of selected serum carotenoids (alpha carotene, beta carotene, lycopene, zeaxanthin, and beta cryptoxanthin) are associated with an increased risk of CIN. In a recent study of 241 southwestern American Indian women, 81 with diagnosed CIN II/III were compared to 160 women with normal cervical epithelium. After adjusting for confounding factors, there appeared to be a significant association between decreasing serum carotenoid concentrations and increased risk of CIN, particularly the carotenoids beta cryptoxanthin, lutein, and zeaxanthin.

DOSAGE: *75,000 IU twice daily for treatment or 25,000–50,000 IU for prevention of mixed natural carotenes*

## Vitamin B12 - Methylcobalamin

Vitamin B12, B6 and folic acid help to decrease homocysteine levels. When elevated, homocysteine has been associated with an increased risk of cervical cancer. Methylcobalamin is the preferred form of B12 as it is utilized more efficiently in the body.

DOSAGE: *1000 mcg daily*

## Vitamin E – Mixed Tocopherols

Vitamin E is a potent antioxidant and low levels of this vitamin have been associated with an increased risk of all stages of CIN and cervical cancer. Supplementing with vitamin E to produce adequate serum levels is associated with a decreased risk. Vitamin E also promotes tissue healing.

DOSAGE: *400–800 IU daily*

## Selenium – L- Selenomethionine

Selenium is another important antioxidant that protects against many cancers including cervical cancer. It is an important mineral for activating optimal immune functioning. L-selenomethionine is more bioavailable and more easily absorbed in the gastrointestinal tract.

DOSAGE: *200–400 mcg daily*

## Zinc

Zinc is another important immune-building mineral. It also helps with the healing of tissue.

DOSAGE: *30 mg daily*

## Flaxseed Oil and/or Pure Fish Oil

Essential fatty acids in the form of flaxseed or uncontaminated fish oil decrease the formation of PGE2, a type of prostaglandin that acts as a messenger molecule to promote inflammatory pathways in the body. Prostaglandins are made by every one of our cells and can either feed pathways that create disease or restore health. Some prostaglandins can actually inhibit cancer growth and support healthy immune function while others promote cancer. Omega-3s found in fish and flax oil support the "healthy" prostaglandin pathways, preventing disease and abnormal cell growth.

DOSAGE: *Take up to 2 tbsp of flax oil daily and/or up to 3000 mg fish oil daily with a minimum of 1000 mg EPA and 600 mg DHA.*

## Probiotics – *Lactobacillus acidophilus and Bifidobacterium spp.*

Probiotics are known to have an important role in the maintenance of normal flora in the gastrointestinal tract. They are also essential for the detoxification of excess estrogens from the body through the bowel along with adequate dietary fibre. Women with CIN I or II have altered estrogen metabolism and have higher 16alpha hydroxyestrone, a potent carcinogen, and fewer 2-hydroxyestrone metabolites that are protective. Probiotics also support optimal immune function as 70% of our immune cells do reside in our gut!

DOSAGE: *at least 10 billion CFU daily with food*

## Green Tea Extract

Green tea has recently been shown to prevent and/or treat HPV-related lesions. Epigallocatechin-3-gallate (EGCG) inhibits cervical cell proliferation and induces cell death (apoptosis) for cancer cells. It therefore possesses anti-tumour effects.

DOSAGE: *300 mg daily, take **EstroSense®**, which combines green tea extract amongst other important anti-cancer nutrients.*

## Indole-3-Carbinol (I3C)

Indole-3-carbinol is a chemical compound that is found in cruciferous vegetables, including cabbage, broccoli, Brussels sprouts, cauliflower and kale. I3C has been shown to prevent abnormal cell growth and tumour progression. I3C increases the protective 2-hydroxyestrones without increasing the other harmful estrogens.

DOSAGE: *300 mg daily, take **EstroSense®**, which combines I3C amongst many other important anti-cancer nutrients.*

## Liver Support – *EstroSense®*

EstroSense is a unique formula that combines indole-3-carbinol, DIM, calcium-d-glucarate, sulforaphane, milk thistle and potent anti-cancer antioxidants (curcumin, rosemary extract, lycopene, green tea extract) to help maintain healthy hormone levels by targeting estrogen metabolism. This may be helpful in CIN II and III as well as other estrogen-related cancers such as breast, uterine and ovarian.

CIN II and III have been shown to have altered estrogen metabolism with higher levels of 16alpha hydroxyestrone (a carcinogen) and fewer

2-hydroxyestrone (protective) metabolites than normal.

DOSAGE: *3 capsules twice daily*

## CONVENTIONAL MEDICINE

### Loop Electrosurgical Excision Procedure (LEEP) Treatment
This procedure involves using electro-surgery to remove the diseased tissue from the cervix. This is the most common treatment.

### Cryotherapy
This procedure is used for small and mild lesions and involves using liquid nitrogen to freeze the affected cervical tissue. The frozen tissue dies, breaks down and is discharged from the body.

### Laser Surgery
This procedure involves a narrow beam of laser light to kill abnormal cells.

### Hysterectomy
In advanced cases of cervical cancer, a hysterectomy is performed (removal of cervix and uterus) and radiation may be recommended.

### HPV Vaccine
Two vaccines are available to prevent the human papillomavirus (HPV) types that cause most cervical cancers. These vaccines are Cervarix and Gardasil. One of the HPV vaccines, Gardasil, also prevents genital warts, as well as anal, vulvar and vaginal cancers. Both vaccines are given in three shots over six months.

There has been controversy regarding the HPV vaccine. Women of all ages are encouraged to do their research before deciding on the vaccine.

Some reported side effects include: fainting, nausea, fever, headaches, blood clots, and neurological disorders.

--------- CHAPTER 6 ---------

# CYSTITIS – BLADDER INFECTION

Urinary tract infections (UTIs) are responsible for more than seven million visits to physician offices per year and are the second-most common type of infection in the body. Infections of the lower urinary tract (urethra and bladder) are surprisingly most common in young women, during pregnancy and in peri- and postmenopausal women.

One in five women will develop a UTI some time during her lifetime.

UTIs can chronically recur – women with a history of recurrent urinary tract infections will typically have an episode at least once every year.

Chronic urinary tract infections can pose significant problems for some women since 55% of infections can eventually involve the upper urinary tract – the kidneys. Another problem with chronic UTIs is the potential for antibiotic resistance. Many women are on antibiotics more often than off, causing disruption and imbalance in natural bacteria flora. Although UTIs are not as common in men (except in infants), they can indicate an obstruction such as a stone or an enlarged prostate and therefore, are uncommon in men under the age of 50.

## SIGNS and SYMPTOMS
Although some UTIs can be asymptomatic, most present with the

following signs and symptoms:

- A strong, persistent urge to urinate
- A burning sensation when urinating
- Passing frequent, small amounts of urine
- Blood in the urine
- Passing milky, cloudy or strong-smelling urine
- Discomfort in the pelvic area, even when not urinating
- A feeling of pressure in the lower abdomen
- Low-grade fever.

## CAUSES

The urinary system consists of the kidneys, ureters, bladder and urethra. This system and its parts play a role in removing waste from the body. The kidneys – a pair of bean-shaped organs located in the back of your upper abdomen – filter waste from the blood and regulate concentrations of many substances. Tubes called ureters carry urine from the kidneys to the bladder, where it's stored until it exits your body through the urethra.

When the kidneys secrete urine, it is sterile until it reaches the urethra, which transports it from the bladder to the urethral opening. UTIs typically occur when bacteria outside the body enter the urinary tract through the urethra and begin to multiply. The urinary system is designed to keep out these microscopic invaders by the following defenses: urine flow tends to wash away bacteria; the bladder secretes a protective coating that prevents bacteria from attaching to its wall; the pH of urine has antibacterial properties that inhibit the growth of bacteria; in men the prostatic fluid has many antimicrobial substances; and the body quickly secretes white cells to control the bacteria.

Although bacterial infections are the most common cause of UTIs, a number of non-infectious factors may cause the bladder to become inflamed. Some examples include:

- **Interstitial cystitis** is most commonly diagnosed in women. It can be called "painful bladder syndrome" because of chronic bladder inflammation (see **Interstitial Cystitis** Chapter).

- **Drug-induced cystitis.** Some medications, particularly the chemotherapy drugs cyclophosphamide and ifosfamide, can cause inflammation in the bladder as the drug is broken down and exited from the body.
- **Radiation cystitis.** Radiation treatment of the pelvic area can cause inflammatory changes in the bladder tissue.
- **Foreign-body cystitis.** Long-term use of a catheter can predispose the bladder to infections and tissue damage, both of which can cause inflammation.
- **Chemical cystitis.** Some may have hypersensitivities to chemicals contained in certain products such as soaps, feminine hygiene sprays or spermicidal jellies and may develop an allergic-type reaction within the bladder, causing inflammation.
- **Cystitis associated with other conditions.** Cystitis may occur as a complication of other disorders such as gynecological cancers, pelvic inflammatory disorders, endometriosis, Crohn's disease, diverticulitis, lupus and tuberculosis.

## RISK FACTORS

One key reason why women are more likely than men to develop bladder infections or recurrent UTIs is physical anatomy. Women have a shorter urethra which shortens the distance bacteria must travel to reach the bladder. Other factors associated with an increased risk of a bladder infection include:

- **Sexual intercourse** can result in bacteria being pushed into the urethra.
- **Certain types of birth control** such as the use of diaphragms have been found to have an increased risk when compared to other forms of birth control. Using condoms with spermicidal foam is also known to be associated with an increase in UTIs in women.
- **Being Pregnant** can double the incidence of UTIs due to hormonal changes.

- **Menopause** can change the lining of the vagina and women will lose the protective effects of estrogen that decrease the likelihood of UTIs.
- **Contamination from the rectum.** A large number of bacteria live in the rectal area and also on the skin. Bacteria may get into the urine from the urethra and travel into the bladder. Always remember to wipe from front to back!
- **Prolonged use of bladder catheters.** These tubes may be needed in people with chronic illnesses or in older adults. Prolonged use can result in increased vulnerability to bacterial infections as well as bladder tissue damage.
- **A depressed immune system** can put many people at higher risk for UTIs because of a reduced ability to fight off infections. This can occur with conditions such as diabetes, HIV infection, cancer treatments and others.
- **Interference with the flow of urine.** This can occur in conditions such as a stone or tumour in the bladder, strictures or in men, an enlarged prostate.
- **Food allergies/intolerances.** Certain foods can aggravate the bladder and contribute to a depressed immune system causing some to be at higher risk of developing recurrent UTIs.

## TESTS and DIAGNOSIS

In general, diagnosis is made based on the above signs and symptoms and urinary findings.

Microscopic examination of the infected urine will show high levels of white blood cells and bacteria. Culturing the urine will indicate the quantity and type of bacteria involved. The Escherichia coli, or E. Coli bacteria is responsible for 90% of bladder infections. Normally, a UTI does not cause a fever if it is in the bladder or urethra. A fever may indicate that the infection has reached the kidneys.

Other symptoms of a kidney infection include:
- Pain in the back or side, below the ribs

- Nausea and vomiting
- Fever and chills.

## PREVENTION and TREATMENT – Dietary and Lifestyle

### FOOD FACTORS

For most UTIs, a natural approach can be the best treatment and the infection usually resolves quickly without recurrence or complications. There is some concern that antibiotic treatment actually promotes recurrent infections by disturbing healthy bacterial flora of the vagina and increasing antibiotic-resistant strains of E.coli.

One of the primary goals in the natural approach to prevention and treatment of urinary tract infections is to enhance the individual's internal defenses by supporting the immune system.

Increasing urinary flow by drinking adequate amounts of liquids (water, herbal teas, fresh fruit and vegetable juices diluted with at least an equal amount of water) can help flush the urinary tract thus preventing the colonization of bacteria. During a bladder infection, 1.5 to 2 litres or more of liquids should be consumed, with at least half of this amount being plain, filtered water. Concentrated fruit juices with high sugar content, coffee, soft drinks and alcohol should be avoided.

A diet high in refined carbohydrates (breads, pasta, pastries containing sugars in the form of glucose, high fructose corn syrup and sucrose) can significantly reduce the ability of white blood cells to destroy foreign particles and bad bacteria. Since white blood cells play a major role in the defense mechanism against infection, impairment of their activity can lead to an immune-compromised state thus increasing the risk of UTIs.

Optimal immune function can also be enhanced by:

- Increasing the intake of fruits and vegetables. Consume at least eight servings daily especially those from the brassica family (cabbage, broccoli and kale) as well as onions, garlic, leeks, sprouts and sea vegetables. Foods high in beta-carotene are protective and enhance the immune system and include orange fruits and vegetables and leafy greens.

- Adequate protein intake for supporting proper immune function has been studied extensively. Choose both vegetarian and lean animal protein sources. Vegetarian sources include: organic soy foods (tempeh, tofu, soybeans, miso), legumes, nuts and seeds. Fish, eggs, organic and antibiotic/hormone free chicken, turkey and lamb can be rotated weekly and organic lean beef should not be consumed more than once a week.
- Avoid/limit common allergenic foods such as dairy, gluten, eggs, peanuts, and corn as these foods can weaken immune function. Consider allergy testing with your Naturopathic doctor.
- Supporting the adrenal glands – Stress can force the adrenal glands to work harder, increasing hormones such as epinephrine and cortisol. When these hormones are released in excessive amounts, white blood cell formation is inhibited leading to significant immune suppression increasing susceptibility to infection.

## LIFESTYLE TIPS
- Wipe from front to back to prevent bacteria around the anus from entering the vagina or urethra. Use unscented and unbleached toilet paper as many women react to the dyes and chemicals in other toilet papers.
- Don't delay urinating. Holding in urine and not emptying your bladder completely can increase the risk of UTIs.
- Urinating before and after sexual intercourse may decrease the risk of UTIs because it flushes out any bacteria that were introduced during intercourse.
- Use cotton underwear.
- Avoid feminine hygiene deodorants, douches and powders that can lead to irritation of the urethra.
- Only use natural cotton sanitary napkins and tampons.
- Take showers instead of baths.

## KEY SUPPLEMENTS

### Cranberry – *Vaccinium macrocarpon*

Women have used cranberry as a home remedy for decades as a treatment for diseases of the urinary tract. Several studies have shown that cranberries and cranberry juice are effective in prevention and treatment of active urinary tract infections. Cranberries and blueberries belong to the *Vaccinium* species which are rich sources of dietary flavonoids, including anthocyanins and proanthocyanidins. It was once thought that cranberry helped UTIs because of its ability to acidify the urine and the antibacterial effects of hippuric acid, a component of cranberries. However, a clearer understanding of the development of UTIs explains the mechanism or action of cranberries as an anti-adhesion agent preventing bacteria from attaching to the lining of the bladder and urethra.

Cranberries have been found effective in the form of pure juice, capsules and tableted extracts. It should be noted that most cranberry juices sold in the grocery store contain 1/3 cranberry juice, mixed with water and sugar. Remember that sugar has a detrimental effect on immune function and therefore, sweetened cranberry juice is not recommended.

Fresh organic cranberry or organic blueberry juice is preferred or cranberry extracts in pill form.

DOSAGE: *500 mg one to three times daily in capsule form or 250–500 ml of organic fresh cranberry juice daily.*

### D-Mannose

D-Mannose is a simple sugar that prevents adherence of certain bacterial strains to the urinary tract lining. Since the bacteria cannot stick, they are eliminated with normal urination. D-Mannose also appears to support the integrity of the bladder's mucosal lining, which may benefit those suffering from interstitial cystitis.

DOSAGE: *500 mg two to four times daily.*

## Probiotics – *Lactobacillus acidophilus and Bifidobacterium spp*

A number of probiotics have been studied for effectiveness in prevention of recurrent UTIs. Because E.coli, the primary pathogen involved in UTIs, travels from the intestines and/or vagina to inhabit the normally sterile urinary tract, improving the gut or vaginal flora can greatly impact the health of the urinary tract. *Lactobacillus and Bifidobacterium spp.* are common probiotics that help support healthy gut flora and improve immune function.

DOSAGE: *at least 10 billion CFU daily with food.*

****All the above ingredients are found in* **UriSense**®, *which is an excellent product for preventing and treating urinary tract infections.*

DOSAGE: *two to four capsules daily.*

## Uva ursi - *Arctostaphylos uva ursi*

Uva ursi, also known as bearberry is one of the most useful herbs for most cases of UTIs. Much of the research on Uva ursi has focussed on its antiseptic and antibacterial component, arbutin. Uva ursi has been reported to be especially active against E.coli as well as having diuretic properties.

DOSAGE: *250–500 mg three times daily for acute urinary tract infection. It is best not taken daily, long term.*

## Berberine

Berberine is a plant alkaloid with a long history of medicinal use in both Ayurvedic and Chinese medicine. It is present in many plants, including Goldenseal (*Hydrastis canadensis*), Oregon grape (*Berberis aquifolium*) and Barberry (*Berberis vulgaris*). Berberine extracts have demonstrated significant antimicrobial activity against a variety of organisms, including bacteria, viruses, fungi, protozoans, helminthes and Chlamydia.

DOSAGE: *500 mg two to three times daily (in the forms of Goldenseal, Oregon grape and Barberry).*

## Vitamin C

Vitamin C is well known for its immune enhancing properties. In a single-blind trial, 110 pregnant women were divided into two groups: one group received ferrous sulfate, folic acid and 100 mg vitamin C daily, while the other group received only ferrous sulfate and folic acid. The occurrence of UTIs was significantly lower in the group receiving the vitamin C.

DOSAGE: *1000 mg one to four times daily or to bowel tolerance.*

## CONVENTIONAL MEDICINE

### Bio-identical Hormones - Estriol cream or Intravaginal Estriol

As mentioned above, hormonal changes (reduced levels of estrogen) in postmenopausal women result in thinning of the vaginal and urethral tissue, disruption of the normal vaginal flora and an increased risk for UTIs.

In fact, 10-15% of women over the age of 60 suffer from recurrent UTIs. Estriol cream applied nightly can greatly reduce the incidence of UTIs.

### Antibiotics

Antibiotics are typically used to treat urinary tract infections. The type of antibiotic prescribed depends on a health history and the type of bacteria found in the urine.

Antibiotics commonly prescribed for simple urinary tract infections include:
- Sulfamethoxazole-trimethoprim (Bactrim)
- Amoxicillin

- Nitrofurantoin (Macrobid)
- Ciprofloxacin (Cipro).

CHAPTER 7

# ENDOMETRIOSIS

Endometriosis is one of the most common gynecological diseases, affecting more than 5.5 million women in North America alone. It commonly occurs between the ages of 25 and 40 in menstruating women but can occur at a younger age. In some cases, symptoms begin with the onset of menstruation while with others, they develop later, becoming progressively worse until menopause. The most common symptoms of endometriosis are: dysmenorrhea (pain with menstrual cycle), dyspareunia (pain with vaginal intercourse) and infertility. For those women who experience pain as a symptom, it can be so intense that it can affect a woman's quality of life, from her relationships, to her day-to-day activities. Some women don't have any symptoms from endometriosis and others may not find out they have the disease until they have trouble getting pregnant. About 30 to 40% of women with endometriosis are infertile, making it one of the top three causes for female infertility.

Endometriosis occurs when the tissue that normally lines the inside of the uterus – the endometrium – grows outside your uterus. Endometriosis most commonly develops on the ovaries, fallopian tubes, vagina, peritoneum, cervix, behind and around the uterus, bladder or bowels. In extremely rare cases, endometriosis can develop in the lungs or other parts of the body.

In endometriosis, the displaced endometrial tissue continues to act as it normally would during a woman's menstrual cycle - it thickens, breaks down and bleeds with each monthly cycle. Since the displaced tissue has no way to exit the body, it becomes trapped causing irritation, inflammation and pain and leading to the development of scar tissue and adhesions.

## SIGNS and SYMPTOMS

Common signs and symptoms of endometriosis may include (but are not limited to):

- Extremely painful or disabling menstrual cramps (dysmenorrhea) – pain/cramping can occur before, during, or between menses
- Chronic pelvic pain (including low back and pelvic area)
- Pain during or after intercourse
- Painful bowel movements or painful urination during menstrual periods
- Intestinal pain
- Heavy menstrual periods
- Premenstrual spotting or bleeding between menstrual periods
- Infertility
- Other symptoms may include – fatigue, diarrhea, constipation, bloating or nausea, especially during the menstrual period.

 **FACT – Did You Know?**
Abdominal and bowel symptoms linked to endometriosis are commonly misdiagnosed as Irritable Bowel Syndrome (IBS).

## CAUSES

### *Retrograde Flow*

One theory proposed by Sampson in 1927, investigated the process of retrograde flow during menstruation as an explanation for endometriosis. In retrograde menstruation, menstrual blood containing endometrial cells flows back through the fallopian tubes and into the pelvic cavity instead of out of the body. These displaced cells stick to the pelvic walls and surfaces of the pelvic organs, where they grow and continue to thicken and bleed over the course of the menstrual cycle. The problem with this theory is that 90% of menstruating women will have some degree of retrograde flow without endometriosis.

## *Genetics*

Another theory involves genes and embryological origin. Some propose that the disease could be inherited or result from genetic errors, making some women more predisposed to develop the condition than others. Some researchers also believe that the implants may be pieces of the uterus left behind during development which, when activated, secrete chemicals causing nearby capillaries to bleed.

## *Estrogen Dominance*

There is also the theory of estrogen dominance. Estrogen appears to promote the growth of endometriosis and therefore, research is looking into the role of the endocrine system and environmental toxins that mimic estrogen called xenoestrogens.

Studies done on Rhesus monkeys exposed to long-term high dioxin levels have helped identify this concept of xenoestrogens and how they disrupt hormone metabolism. Extensive clinical research links toxins such as PCBs, BPA, plastics, detergents, household cleaners and beauty products to mimicking estrogen in the body thus contributing to estrogen dominance.

## *The Role of the Liver*

The liver is one of the most important organs in the human body because it is involved in the removal of harmful toxins. Because of its key role in detoxification, the liver has an enormous task of breaking down estrogen and eliminating its harmful metabolites through the bile and large intestine.

If the liver is not functioning optimally, poor metabolism of estrogen can result in liver damage and continual recycling of estrogens throughout the body. Since the liver is involved in breaking down 80 to 90% of the hormones in the body, it is imperative that the liver has adequate nutritional and herbal support for optimal functioning.

### The Role of the Gut

A delicate balance between "good" and "bad" bacteria is vitally important for proper hormone and estrogen metabolism.

To eliminate estrogen from the body, the liver inactivates estrogen by attaching a compound called glucaronic acid. Some bad bacteria in the large intestine will secrete an enzyme called beta-glucaronidase that will break off the glucaronic acid thereby releasing the activated stronger estrogen back into the body. These bad bacteria usually feed off unhealthy fats from a poor diet. Proper balance can be restored by increasing good bacteria in the gut by adding *Lactobacillus acidophilus* and *Bifidobacterium* to the diet. This ensures that a higher amount of the inactivated estrogen is able to be eliminated through the large intestine, preventing reactivation and the recycling of stronger bad estrogens throughout the body.

 **FACT – Did You Know?**
Several practitioners have observed that some patients with endometriosis experience improvement of symptoms after going on an anti-candida diet.

### The Immune System

Women with low immune function may be more susceptible to tissue implants and growth due to free radical production versus women with a stronger, balanced immune system.

Natural killer cells are cells of the immune system that help keep tumour and abnormal cell growth in check. There have been studies that suggest a correlation between high levels of estrogen (namely estradiol) and a decreased natural killer cell activity in women with endometriosis.

Another interesting finding is higher levels of antibodies in those women with endometriosis, specifically immunoglobulins IgM and IgG.

Immunoglobulins are part of the immune system and provide protection to the body from foreign toxins. Higher amounts of IgM and IgG can cause destruction of the body's own tissue, attacking their own ovaries and endometrial cells. Some women with endometriosis will also have an autoimmune disease.

### FACT – Did You Know?

Many practitioners report the association between food sensitivities and endometriosis, specifically wheat, dairy, refined sugars, caffeine and alcohol.

## RISK FACTORS

- A mother or sister with endometriosis
- Not having given birth
- A history of pelvic infection
- Menstrual cycles that are shorter than 25 days
- Menstrual periods that are longer than 7 days
- Estrogen dominance
- Hormone replacement therapy
- Exposure to environmental estrogens – dioxin and PCBs (ingested in fish meat, dairy) as well as BPA and phthalates
- Increased body fat
- Diet high in animal fat (increases arachinonic acid, increasing inflammation and pain)
- Lack of exercise from an early age
- Use of IUD
- High stress levels and poor adaptation to stress
- Alcohol use
- Childhood sexual abuse
- Prenatal exposure to high estrogen levels
- Poor liver function
- Bowel toxicity and constipation
- Dysbiosis – imbalance in bowel flora

**FACT – Did You Know?**

One study actually found that women with natural red hair colour are at a higher risk for the development of endometriosis.

## TESTING AND DIAGNOSIS

The diagnosis of endometriosis often begins with a thorough medical history including the description of symptoms, location of pain and when it occurs.

A physical/pelvic exam usually reveals one or more of the following:

- Tenderness of the pelvic area
- Enlarged or tender ovaries
- A uterus that tips backwards and lacks mobility
- Fixed pelvic structures
- Adhesions.

An ultrasound can be useful in identifying cysts associated with endometriosis but won't definitively diagnose endometriosis.

This can only be accomplished during a minor surgical procedure called a laparoscopy.

During a laparoscopy, the surgeon inserts a small viewing instrument with a light (laparoscope) through a small incision in the abdomen. By doing this procedure, a diagnosis can be made based on the characteristic appearance of endometriosis. This can then be further confirmed by doing a biopsy.

### PREVENTION and TREATMENT – Dietary and Lifestyle

## FOOD FACTORS

Endometriosis is a complex disease involving a number of systems in the body. Optimal nutrition to enhance the immune system, balance hormones and help the liver break down environmental and naturally-occurring estrogens, are key approaches in the treatment and prevention of endometriosis.

Research shows that women with endometriosis require more antioxidants from food and supplements. In one study, the diets of women with endometriosis were lower in antioxidants compared to women who didn't have the disease. Some research suggests that free radicals may play a role in allowing endometriosis to grow. As well, due to the increased oxidative stress of endometriosis, the need for antioxidants intensifies.

Enjoy a diet of 50% or more raw fruits and vegetables of all colours to benefit from an ample supply of energy-promoting enzymes.

High fibre foods help support a healthy intestinal tract as well as an optimal balance of "good" to "bad" bacteria. Ensuring an adequate amount of good bacterial flora in the digestive tract helps metabolize excess bad estrogens and prevents the recycling of these estrogens back throughout the body. Up to 30% of women with endometriosis also have gastrointestinal disorders such as constipation. Increasing fibre sources such as psyllium, ground flax, inulin, oat bran, and fruits and vegetables, will help optimize bowel elimination (see **Appendix**).

A diet higher in red meat, pork, dairy, shellfish and peanuts will increase arachidonic acid levels in the body promoting inflammation and pain. By increasing vegetable protein intake with legumes, organic soy, almond and other nut butters and fish, the anti-inflammatory pathways are stimulated, inhibiting tumour growth and possibly endometrial growth.

Other foods that will increase arachidonic acid and thus inflammation are caffeine, alcohol, chocolate and sugar.

Certain foods will enhance liver function and therefore, improve detoxification of harmful estrogen metabolites and toxins. This can prevent estrogen dominance. Some liver-friendly foods to include in the diet are broccoli, kale, cabbage, artichokes, garlic, parsley, celery, beets and beet greens, dandelion greens, and turmeric.

**FACT – Did You Know?**

A prospective study showed that women with the highest intake of omega-3 fatty acids were 22% less likely to be diagnosed with endometriosis than women with the lowest intake levels.

## LIFESTYLE TIPS

- Use castor oil packs before bed several times a week to improve pelvic circulation, soften adhesions and reduce pain (see **Appendix** – *Castor Oil Pack*)

   *\*Do not use castor oil packs during menstruation or if pregnant.*

- Regular, moderate exercise is recommended to improve circulation, increase endorphins, decrease circulating estrogen and decrease pain.

- Use relaxation techniques such as meditation, yoga or breathing exercises to lower stress.

- Buy only non-bleached feminine products, toilet paper and tissues to reduce your exposure to dioxins.

- Eliminate xenoestrogens from the home, store food in glass, not plastic; drink water out of glass and avoid cans lined with plastic to reduce exposure to BPA (bisphenol-A). Avoid cosmetics, shampoo, toothpaste and other beauty products containing parabens.

### *Body/Mind Connection*

Endometriosis is associated with disappointment and frustration. Focus on feeling fulfilled.

## KEY SUPPLEMENTS

### Liver Support – *EstroSense*®

Endometriosis is linked to estrogen dominance and therefore, supporting healthy liver function and detoxification lessens the burden of excess estrogens on the body and prevents endometriosis. *EstroSense*® contains the herbs milk thistle, indole-3-carbinol, DIM, sulforaphane and calcium-d-glucarate that help with the break down of these harmful estrogens. As well, it provides antioxidant support with lycopene, rosemary and green tea extract for removal of any toxic by-products.

DOSAGE: *3 capsules twice daily*

## Vitamin C
Vitamin C decreases pelvic pain by decreasing oxidative stress, which is elevated in women with endometriosis. Vitamin C also supports healthy immunity and decreases capillary fragility and tumour growth.

DOSAGE: *2000-6000 mg in divided doses daily or to bowel tolerance*

## Vitamin E
Vitamin E helps decrease pelvic pain and inflammation by decreasing oxidative stress and supports healthy immunity.

DOSAGE: *400-800 IU daily*

***Note: Other antioxidants that may benefit endometriosis include: zinc, selenium, alpha-lipoic acid, and beta-carotene.*

## Vitamin B Complex
B Vitamins help support the liver and improve the metabolism of harmful estrogens.

DOSAGE: *50-100 mg daily*

## Pure Fish Oil- Omega-3 Fatty Acids
Essential fatty acids in the form of uncontaminated pure fish oil block the formation of PGE2 which is a messenger molecule that helps increase inflammatory pathways in the body. They are very helpful in reducing pain and inflammation and help to prevent additional endometrial growth.

DOSAGE: *3000 mg fish oil daily with a minimum of 1000 mg EPA and 600 mg DHA.*

## Chaste Tree Berry - *Vitex agnus castus*

Chaste Tree Berry (Vitex) is one of the single most important herbs for supporting hormonal imbalance in women. The effect of chaste tree is on the hypothalamus/hypophysis axis in which it increases luteinizing hormone and has an effect which favours progesterone. This action prevents excess estrogen from stimulating endometrial tissue.

DOSAGE: *Take up to 400 mg daily.*
*\*It may take up to three months to see results.*

## Calcium/Magnesium

Calcium and magnesium help relax muscles and cramping that may be associated with endometriosis.

DOSAGE: *1000 mg of calcium citrate/malate and 500 mg of magnesium bisglycinate/citrate*

## Probiotics – *Lactobacillus acidophilus* and *Bifidobacterium spp.*

Probiotics are known to play an important role in the maintenance of normal flora in the gastrointestinal tract. They also help with the detoxification and binding of harmful estrogens in the digestive tract and eliminate them from the body through the colon.

DOSAGE: *at least 10 billion CFU daily with food.*

## Natural Bio-Identical Progesterone Cream

Women who are deficient in progesterone often have estrogen excess. Natural progesterone may be helpful in reducing painful cramping and uterine contractions.

DOSAGE: *Take ¼-1/2 tsp twice daily from Day 10 to Day 26*

## CONVENTIONAL TREATMENT

Conventional treatment for endometriosis is usually with medications or surgery. The approach chosen will depend on the severity of symptoms and whether the woman hopes to become pregnant. Doctors generally recommend conservative treatment first, opting for surgery as a last resort.

### Pain medications

For mild or moderate pain, usually over-the-counter pain medications are recommended such as ibuprofen (Advil or Motrin), naproxen or mefenamic acid to help ease painful menstrual cramps.

### Hormone therapy

Supplementing with hormones is sometimes effective in reducing or eliminating the pain of endometriosis. This may involve manipulating hormone levels because rise and fall of hormones during a woman's menstrual cycle can cause endometrial implants to thicken, break down and bleed. These methods include:

- Oral contraceptives
- Gonadotropin-releasing hormone analogs which block the production of ovarian-stimulating hormones. This prevents menstruation and dramatically lowers estrogen levels, causing endometrial implants to shrink. These drugs create an artificial menopause that can sometimes lead to side effects such as hot flashes and vaginal dryness.
- Danazol is another drug that blocks the production of ovarian-stimulating hormones, preventing menstruation and the symptoms of endometriosis. In addition, it suppresses the growth of the endometrium. However, danazol may not be the first choice because it can cause unwanted side effects, such as acne and facial hair.

### Conservative surgery

Conservative surgery involves the removal of endometrial growth, scar tissue and adhesions without removing the reproductive organs. The specialist usually performs this procedure using a laparoscope, a small viewing instrument inserted through an incision near the navel. The doctor then inserts other instruments through another incision to remove endometrial implanted tissue using laser surgery or electrocautery (burning).

## Hysterectomy

In severe cases of endometriosis, surgery to remove the uterus and cervix (total hysterectomy) as well as both ovaries, may be the best treatment. Hysterectomy alone is not effective - the estrogen your ovaries produce can stimulate any remaining endometriosis and cause pain to persist. Surgery is typically considered a last resort, especially for women still in their reproductive years.

-------------------- CHAPTER 8 --------------------

# FIBROCYSTIC BREASTS

Formerly referred to as fibrocystic breast disease, fibrocystic breasts are characterized by lumpiness and discomfort in one or both breasts. Affecting more than 60% of women, it tends to be an issue for women primarily between the ages of 30 and 50, with impact diminishing after menopause.

Monthly hormone fluctuations are the most significant contributing factor to fibrocystic breasts as a woman's body prepares each month for a possible pregnancy. The critical hormones estrogen and progesterone, directly affect breast tissue by causing cells to grow and multiply. Prolactin, growth factor, insulin and thyroid hormone are also involved.

During the monthly cycle, hormones stimulate the growth of breast glandular tissues and increase the activity of blood vessels, cell metabolism and supporting tissue in anticipation of pregnancy. If pregnancy doesn't occur, breast cells undergo programmed cell death (apoptosis). Cells are devoured by enzymes and inflammatory scavenger cells. The inflammation may lead to scarring (fibrosis) of breast tissue. The efficiency of this cleanup process can vary from one woman to another and even be different within a breast.

Over time, from puberty to menopause, the repeated monthly hormonal cycles and the accumulation of fluid, cells, and cellular debris within the breast can lead to fibrocystic breasts. After menopause, fibrocystic breast disease tends to be less of a problem. Although benign, fibrocystic breasts can confound the detection of breast cancer.

## SIGNS AND SYMPTOMS

While symptoms of fibrocystic breast disease vary among women and even between one woman's breasts, common indications include breast tenderness or pain; lumpiness in one or both breasts; nipple itching; and the feeling of breast heaviness. Some women will describe their breast lumps or "cysts" as soft, tender, and moveable. The symptoms can be intermittent, coming and going with the monthly cycle, or persistent throughout the month. Diagnosis can be challenging if, for example, there are no symptoms and neither the woman nor her doctor can detect lumps. In other women, lumps are easily located throughout both breasts.

## CAUSES

Women with irregular menstrual cycles seem to suffer more severe fibrocystic breasts as time goes on, likely because of the prolonged and irregular hormonal stimulation of the breasts. Symptoms also tend to be the most severe right before the menstrual period due to an increased estrogen to progesterone ratio leading to an estrogen dominance picture. Other causes include:

- An underactive or low thyroid as this may cause elevated prolactin levels
- An iodine deficiency which would cause the cells in the breast tissue to be more sensitive to estrogen
- Too much estrone and too little estriol, an imbalance in estrogen levels
- Other nutritional deficiencies such as vitamin E, vitamin B6, CoQ10, and essential fatty acids
- Overconsumption of meat, dairy, bad fats
- Heavy metal toxicity specifically lead, cadmium, and mercury
- Accumulation of xenoestrogens in the breast tissue (PCBs, dioxin,

bisphenol-A, phthalates, parabens)
- Bowel toxicity
- Liver toxicity or sluggishness
- Poor lymphatic circulation, possibly from a tight bra with underwiring or lack of exercise
- Consumption of methylxanthine, found in coffee, black tea, cola, chocolate and caffeinated medications.

 **FACT - Did You Know?**

Wearing a bra that is too tight or that has underwiring can affect breast health by compressing lymphatic vessels causing congestion and inflammation in the breast tissue. Choose a bra that fits properly, is not too tight, preferably without underwiring and when removed, does not leave any red marks on the skin.

## TESTING and DIAGNOSIS

### *Breast Self-Examination*
Monthly breast self-exams are important in the detection of any changes that occur in the breasts (see *"Breast Self Examination"* in **Breast Cancer** Chapter). Medical doctors will often perform breast exams as part of an annual physical check-up. During the exam, the doctor visually and manually examines the breasts and the lymph nodes in the lower neck and underarm area for any unusual changes or findings. The lumps in fibrocystic breast disease are typically not attached to overlying or underlying tissue and generally are easiest to locate on the upper breast toward the underarm. Lumps have round, smooth borders and feel somewhat pliable. Sometimes fibrocystic areas feel irregular in shape or like small beads.

### *Ultrasound*
Along with being familiar with your breasts and becoming aware of changes, ultrasound exams are helpful in assessing breast lumps. Women under age 30 might undergo this test instead of mammography because

it can better evaluate dense breast tissue. Ultrasound is also particularly helpful in distinguishing between fluid-filled breast cysts and solid masses.

## *Mammography vs Thermography*

Sometimes, if a woman or health practitioner detects a breast lump or unusual thickening in the breast tissue, mammography may be suggested. Many naturopathic doctors and some complementary medical doctors are now recommending breast thermography as a screening for breast health instead of mammography. Breast thermography is a type of imaging procedure where infrared images of the breast are analyzed and rated to determine the risk of developing breast cancer. It uses infrared sensors to detect heat and increased vascularity in the breast tissue, therefore detecting metabolic activity. Typically in cancerous tumours, there is an ever-increasing need for nutrients. The tumours will often increase circulation to their cells by creating new blood vessels to feed the tumour. This process frequently results in a temperature increase of the breast allowing thermography to detect these heat patterns.

Mammography is a structural imaging technique, meaning that it is ideal for detecting actual structural differences or suspicious lumps but sometimes it may be too late. Breast thermography can be used preventatively as a screening tool and like mammography, if something suspicious is discovered, a tissue biopsy of the breast is always the gold standard for diagnosis of breast cancer.

## PREVENTION and TREATMENT – Dietary and Lifestyle

## FOOD FACTORS

The key to relieving symptoms of fibrocystic breasts is to balance hormones. Increase vegetables from the brassica family which contain compounds that metabolize "bad" estrogens and convert them into friendlier ones. Include foods such as kale, broccoli, cabbage, cauliflower and Brussels sprouts. Support healthy bowel function to help move estrogens out of the digestive tract by consuming a diet that contains adequate fibre (see **Appendix**). Excellent sources of fibre include ground flax, oat bran, psyllium, chia or hemp seeds, legumes and plenty of fruits and vegetables. Flush fibre through the intestines with plenty of water.

Reduce inflammatory foods in the diet by avoiding saturated fats (red meat, dairy), trans fats and sugar. Consume plenty of deep-water fatty fish like anchovies and wild salmon as well as nuts and seeds for sources of anti-inflammatory omega-3 fats and omega-6 fats gamma-linoleic acid (GLA).

Avoid sources of caffeine such as coffee, tea, chocolate and colas. Caffeine, theophylline, and theobromine are known as methylxanthines. These compounds promote the overproduction of fibrous tissue and cysts in the breast tissue, which may be linked to fibrocystic breast disease. In one study, limiting methylxanthines (coffee, tea, colas, chocolate and caffeinated medications) resulted in a 97.5% improvement in breast tissue for the 45 women who completely abstained from the above foods. There was a 75% improvement for the 28 women who only limited their consumption. The women who continued with their consumption showed little improvement.

Choose organic foods whenever possible to reduce exposure to xenoestrogenic pesticides, herbicides and fungicides used in conventional farming.

## LIFESTYLE TIPS

- Book yourself an appointment for a bra fitting. Most women are wearing the wrong size which can lead to spilling over of breast tissue. This can affect circulation, causing breast and shoulder pain and lack of support. Choose a bra that provides adequate support.
- To replace coffee, enjoy herbal teas containing hibiscus flowers, shepherd's purse, raspberry leaves, vitex berries, orange peels and yarrow herbs and flowers to help balance hormones.

> *Body/Mind Connection*
> Breast problems often relate to a refusal to nourish yourself. Strive for balance and nourishment in all aspects of your life.

- Warm heating pads or hot water bottles can help soothe aching breasts.
- Learn to read labels to avoid estrogen-mimicking chemicals in home and beauty care products. (see **Breast Cancer** Chapter)
- Know your breasts! Monthly breast self-exams will help to ease your mind.
- Regular exercise helps to improve lymphatic circulation and promote elimination of toxins.
- Schedule breast thermography at least once a year.

 **FACT – Did You Know?**

Castor oil is an excellent anti-inflammatory when used topically and can be used for improving lymph drainage and detoxification.

Women can apply castor oil to the breasts as well as to the liver three or more times a week. Soak a cloth or old t-shirt with oil, apply to area and then cover with a heating pad. As castor oil is quite messy, be sure to wear clothing that you don't mind getting stained.

Castor oil packs should not be done during menstruation or if pregnant (see *Castor Oil Pack* in **Appendix**).

## KEY SUPPLEMENTS

### Flaxseed Oil and/or Pure Fish Oil

Essential fatty acids in the form of flaxseed or uncontaminated fish oil block the formation of PGE2, which is a messenger molecule that promotes inflammatory pathways in the body. These oils may be beneficial in reducing breast pain and inflammation as well as preventing abnormal changes in the breast tissue.

DOSAGE: *Take up to 2 tbsp of flax oil daily and/or up to 3000 mg fish oil daily with a minimum of 800 mg EPA and 400 mg DHA.*

## Evening Primrose Oil

Fibrocystic breast pain can be alleviated with the use of omega-6s such as evening primrose oil which contains linoleic acid (LA) and gamma linolenic acid (GLA). The body uses LA to produce GLA to help produce beneficial prostaglandins that regulate inflammation, pain, blood pressure, fluid balance and blood clotting. Researchers have investigated the benefits of evening primrose oil for premenstrual breast pain as well as fibrocystic breasts. In one study, 291 women were given three grams of evening primrose oil per day for three to six months. Results showed that almost half of the 92 women with cyclical breast pain experienced improvement, compared to one-fifth of those receiving the placebo. In another study, 73 women received three grams of evening primrose oil or placebo for three months. Pain and tenderness were significantly reduced in both cyclical and noncyclical groups while the women who took the placebo did not improve.

DOSAGE: *1500 mg twice daily*

## Vitamin E

Vitamin E has been shown to relieve many PMS symptoms, particularly fibrocystic breasts. One double blind study was conducted in 150 women in Iran. Two groups of 75 women each were evaluated for length and severity of breast pain measured by a breast pain chart. 200 IU of vitamin E or placebo were given twice daily for four months. Breast pain and duration were evaluated at the end of the second and fourth months. At the end of two months for the vitamin E group, symptoms were dramatically better than placebo in severity and duration. This was reported in about 70% of the women.

DOSAGE: *400-800 IU daily*

## Iodine and the Thyroid

Much research shows that supporting an underactive thyroid results in decreased breast pain and breast nodules and therefore helps with the symptoms of fibrocystic breast disease. It is not known what the exact mechanism of action is, but there is a definite affinity for both thyroid hormone and iodine in the breast tissue. When iodine is deficient, the breast tissue becomes more sensitive to estrogenic stimulation creating estrogen dominance in the breast. Iodine supplementation is also known to have significant anti-inflammatory and antifibrotic effects.

DOSAGE: *150–500 mcg of potassium iodide daily*

## Support the Liver

Since the liver is the primary site for healthy estrogen metabolism and clearance, supporting the liver and its pathways is essential for preventing estrogen dominance in the body as well as the breast tissue. Adequate levels of B vitamins are necessary for estrogen clearance from the body, especially vitamin B6 and folic acid. Other important liver detoxifiers include:

- Calcium D-glucarate
- Indole-3-carbinol
- Milk Thistle extract
- DIM
- Sulforaphane
- Turmeric.

The above herbs help to eliminate excess estrogens from the body through the liver, help metabolize and convert cancer-causing estrogens into non-toxic forms, protect the liver from environmental toxins and inhibit abnormal cell growth in the breast tissue. Antioxidants are essential in the detoxification process as toxin compounds are being broken down and dangerous byproducts are being released. Antioxidants such as green tea extract, rosemary and lycopene help reduce the toxin burden on the body by binding free radicals and other harmful toxins.

*\*\*\*All the above nutrients are found in* **EstroSense®**, *an excellent product for supporting healthy liver detoxification, and reducing symptoms of estrogen dominance such as fibrocystic breasts.*

DOSAGE: *Take 3 capsules twice daily.*

## Vitamin B6 and B complex

As mentioned above vitamin B6 and the other B vitamins are essential in supporting healthy liver detoxification and estrogen metabolism.

DOSAGE: *150–250 mg of Vitamin B6 and 50 mg of a B Complex daily*

## Support the Colon and Digestive tract

There is a strong correlation between breast disease and constipation caused by low fibre in the diet. Women who have less than three bowel movements per week have a 4.5 times greater rate of fibrocystic breast disease than women who have at least one bowel movement a day. The bacteria in the large intestine are key to the removal of excess steroid hormones such as estrogens through the bowel and preventing them from being reabsorbed into the body.

## Probiotics - *Lactobacillus acidophilus* and *Bifidobacterium spp.*

Probiotics are known to play an important role in the maintenance of normal flora in the gastrointestinal tract. They also help with the detoxification and binding of harmful estrogens in the digestive tract and elimination of them from the body through the colon.

DOSAGE: *Take at least 10 billion CFU daily with food.*

## Fibre – *Ultimate FibreLean*™

DOSAGE: *Take one scoop twice daily in water, oatmeal or smoothie.*

## Chaste Tree Berry – *Vitex agnus castus*

Vitex is used to alleviate many gynecological symptoms such as PMS, fibrocystic breasts, PCOS and fibroids, just to name a few. It seems to work in favour of progesterone, reducing symptoms of estrogen dominance and reducing abnormal breast tissue growth and pain.

DOSAGE: *Take up to 400 mg daily.*
*It may take up to three months to see results.*

## CoQ10

Coenzyme Q10 is an important antioxidant and free radical scavenger and may be useful in reducing inflammation and pain associated with fibrocystic breasts.

DOSAGE: *Take up to 200 mg daily.*

## Botanicals

Herbs can be very useful in reducing symptoms of breast pain, swelling and cysts in the breasts. Herbal diuretics such as dandelion leaf (*Taraxacum officinale*) can help reduce swelling in the breasts. Dandelion leaf is preferred over many synthetic diuretics as it does not deplete potassium. Other diuretics to consider are cleavers (*Galium aparine*), yarrow (*Achillea millefolium*) and uva ursi (*Arctostaphylos uva ursi*). Poke root (*Phytolacca americana*) is an herb that can be applied as an oil to the breasts and rubbed in like a lotion to reduce painful lumps or nodules associated with fibrocystic breasts.

## Breast Oil

Mix 20 ml of each:
Phytolacca oil
Calendula oil
Dandelion oil
Red clover oil

Mix in with 150 ml of carrier oil:
Extra virgin olive oil
Almond oil

DOSAGE: *Apply to breast nightly for two weeks then reduce to three times per week.*

### Natural Progesterone Cream

Fibrocystic breasts are partly due to a high estrogen/low progesterone imbalance and many practitioners find using progesterone cream useful in reducing symptoms.

DOSAGE: *Apply ¼ tsp twice per day from Day 15 to Day 27 of the menstrual cycle.*

## CONVENTIONAL MEDICINE

Common medications used for breast pain and fibrocystic breasts include:

- Diuretics – which help reduce swelling by increasing fluid elimination but often deplete potassium.
- Anti-Inflammatories – help with the pain but can be hard on the stomach and liver.
- Synthetic hormone therapy – drugs such as the steroid danazol, which can be effective but may cause facial and body hair growth, deepening of the voice, weight gain, acne, and other side effects. Other drugs include birth control pills, synthetic progestin, tamoxifen and bromocriptene.

CHAPTER 9

# GENITAL HERPES

Genital herpes is a common sexually transmitted disease (STD) caused by either the herpes simplex virus type 1 (HSV-1) or type 2 (HSV-2). HSV-1 is responsible for causing cold sores on the lips, pharynx and cornea and for causing 20% of genital herpes outbreaks. It is typically spread by contact with oral secretions.

HSV-2 is the more common cause of genital herpes and is spread by contact with the sores, usually during sexual activity.

In the U.S., at least 45 million people ages 12 and older have had a genital herpes infection at some time. It is estimated that up to one million new infections occur each year.

Genital herpes infection with HSV-2 is more common in women (almost 1 in 5) than in men (almost 1 in 9). This may be due to the fact that male-to-female transmission is more likely than female–to-male transmission.

## 🔆 FACT – Did You Know?

Research studies show that most people with genital herpes do not realize they are infected; they either have never had any symptoms or have not recognized their symptoms as herpes.

## SIGNS and SYMPTOMS

The symptoms of genital herpes vary from person to person but these can be severe if they occur with the first outbreak. Subsequent outbreaks are typically mild if the strain is HSV-1.

Genital herpes can start off with slight tingling and prickly sensations followed by pain or itching beginning usually within a week after exposure to an infected sexual partner. However, symptoms can start from 1 to 26 days after exposure. Small red bumps or tiny white blisters may appear. The blisters eventually rupture, becoming ulcers that ooze or bleed. Then scabs form and the ulcers heal. In women, sores can erupt in the vaginal area, external genitals, buttocks, anus or cervix. In men, sores can appear on the penis, scrotum, buttocks, anus or thighs or inside the urethra, the tube inside the penis leading to the bladder.

Further symptoms include painful urination, swollen lymph nodes in the groin and flu-like symptoms (headache, muscle aches, fever). There can be pain and tenderness in the genital area until the infection clears.

## RISK FACTORS

The first herpes outbreak is typically the worst. As mentioned above, genital herpes is spread by direct contact with an infected person. Sexual intercourse and oral sex are the most common methods of spreading genital herpes. Other risk factors include:

- Female
- Low education level
- Poverty
- Cocaine use
- A history of two or more lifetime sexual partners
- Unprotected sex
- Having a sexual partner with genital herpes.

Subsequent outbreaks can be caused by various factors including:

- Physical or emotional stress
- Anxiety/depression
- Hormonal changes during a woman's menstrual cycle
- Overexposure to sunlight
- Immune stress/deficiency
- Foods high in arginine
- A deficiency in the amino acid lysine.

## COMPLICATIONS

If genital herpes is not treated or there are repeated flare-ups, other health complications can occur such as:

- *Other sexually transmitted infections.* Having genital sores increases the risk of transmitting or contracting other sexually transmitted infections, including the AIDS virus.
- *Newborn infections.* Babies born to infected mothers can be exposed to the virus during the birthing process. This can result in some cases in brain damage, blindness or death for the newborn. Some medical professionals will recommend a c-section instead of a vaginal birth because of this associated risk.
- *Bladder problems.* In some cases, the erupted sores associated with genital herpes can cause inflammation around the urethra, the tube that delivers urine from the bladder to the outside world. The swelling can close the urethra for several days, requiring the insertion of a catheter to drain the bladder.
- *Meningitis.* In rare cases, an HSV infection can cause inflammation of the membranes and cerebrospinal fluid surrounding the brain and spinal cord.
- *Proctitis (rectal inflammation).* Genital herpes can lead to inflammation of the lining of the rectum, particularly in men who have sex with men.

## TESTING AND DIAGNOSIS

The diagnosis of genital herpes is typically based on the patient's medical history, a physical exam and laboratory tests.

Medical history:

- Pregnancy history
- Types of sexual activity and frequency
- Sexually active with men, women or both
- Birth control method being used, if any
- Knowledge of partner or partners' sexual history
- Use of condoms for protection from sexually transmitted infections.

Laboratory tests:

- A blood test that analyzes a sample of blood for the presence of HSV antibodies to detect a past herpes infection.
- A viral culture that involves taking a tissue sample or scraping of the sores for examination in the lab.

### PREVENTION and TREATMENT – Dietary and Lifestyle

### FOOD FACTORS

A healthy diet packed full of nutritious whole foods is fundamental in keeping the body strong and supporting a resilient immune system.

Reoccurring herpes simplex infections are strongly dependent on how well the immune response is functioning. Consuming large amounts of refined carbohydrates can impair proper immune function.

Some patients have observed that HSV outbreaks do recur after the ingestion of too many sweets. A study published in the *American Journal of Clinical Nutrition* reported that human subjects who were given 75g of glucose, showed significantly depressed immune function within 30 to 60 minutes of ingestion. The direct correlation between refined carbohydrate intake and the susceptibility to an HSV outbreak has not been investigated. But based on research describing the impact of refined carbohydrates on the immune system, it makes good sense to limit their intake.

Immune-boosting strategies include:

- Increase the intake of fruits and vegetables. Consume at least eight servings daily especially those from the brassica family (cabbage, broccoli, and kale), as well as onions, garlic, leeks, sprouts and sea vegetables. Foods high in beta-carotene (orange fruits and vegetables, leafy greens) enhance the immune system.
- Ensure adequate protein intake from both vegetarian and lean animal protein sources. Vegetarian sources include: organic soy foods (tempeh, tofu, soybeans, miso), legumes, nuts and seeds. Fish, eggs, organic chicken, turkey and lamb can be rotated weekly and organic lean beef should not be consumed more than once a week.
- Avoid/limit common allergenic foods such as dairy, gluten, eggs, soy, peanuts, and corn as these foods can weaken immune function.
- Include adequate amounts of fibre such as legumes, ground flax, oat bran, fruits and vegetables (see **Appendix**).
- Minimize refined sugars, carbohydrates and hydrogenated fats.
- Drink at least one litre of water daily.
- Support the adrenal glands. Stress can force the adrenal glands to work harder, increasing hormones such as epinephrine and cortisol. When these hormones are released in excessive amounts, white blood cell formation is inhibited leading to significant immune suppression increasing susceptibility to infection.

## *The Lysine/Arginine Connection*

The herpes simplex virus synthesizes proteins that are rich in the amino acid arginine and low in the amino acid lysine. Arginine is also required for the replication of the herpes virus. Lysine appears to block arginine by several mechanisms: it competes with arginine for reabsorption in the kidneys thereby increasing arginine excretion, it competes with arginine for intestinal absorption, it induces an enzyme that breaks arginine down and competes with arginine for transport into cells.

Extensive research has shown that the herpes virus is dependent on proteins rich in arginine for its replication. Therefore, reducing high arginine foods and increasing high lysine foods can be quite beneficial. The amino acid lysine has antiviral properties that help block arginine and low arginine will suppress the activation of HSV replication.

## Foods HIGH in ARGININE – Reduce these foods to prevent HSV

- Chocolate
- Nuts and seeds: peanuts, almonds, cashews, sunflower seeds, walnuts, pecans, brazil nuts, sesame seeds

## Foods HIGH in LYSINE – Increase these foods to prevent HSV

- Most vegetables
- Fish
- Turkey and chicken
- Legumes

## LIFESTYLE TIPS

- Learn to recognize early signs of an HSV outbreak such as tingling or prickling sensations, or itching so that appropriate treatment can be initiated immediately.
- Refrain from sexual contact during an outbreak.
- Use barrier methods of birth control with new sexual partners or with a previously infected sexual partner. The transmission of HSV can occur even if there are no visible symptoms.
- During an outbreak, the virus can be transferred from one body site to another, so if there is a lesion present, either pat or air-dry after showering and wash towels after a single use.

**FACT - Did You Know?**

Simply applying ice for ten minutes several times daily can limit discomfort and swelling or even keep an outbreak from fully erupting. Do this preferably during the initial stages of itching or tingling or even if the eruption has appeared.

## KEY SUPPLEMENTS

### L-Lysine

A diet high in the amino acid lysine and low in arginine has become an effective treatment for HSV infections and outbreaks.

As mentioned above, lysine has antiviral activity blocking the replication of the Herpes simplex virus.

DOSAGE: *For acute outbreaks, take 1000 mg three times daily and for maintenance take 1000 mg daily.*

### Vitamin C and Bioflavonoids

Vitamin C is known as an important antioxidant to enhance immune function and has been shown to inactivate a wide range of viruses including Herpes simplex. During an acute outbreak, dosing vitamin C to bowel tolerance as high as 5000-6000 mg per day may be considered. For long-term prevention and maintenance 600-3000 mg of vitamin C daily is most reasonable.

DOSAGE: *For acute episodes, take vitamin C to bowel tolerance and for maintenance take 600 – 3000 mg daily (or to bowel tolerance).*

### Zinc

Supplementation with zinc has been shown to reduce the severity and duration of HSV outbreaks. In one study, oral administration of 25 mg of zinc and 250 mg of vitamin C each twice daily for six weeks appeared to reduce the duration and severity of Herpes simplex outbreaks during the supplementation period, especially for patients who experienced sun-induced herpetic outbreaks.

DOSAGE: *25 mg twice daily with food for six weeks during the outbreak then reduce to 25 mg daily as maintenance.*

## Vitamin B12 Injections

A naturopathic doctor or complementary health care provider can administer intramuscular injections of vitamin B12 at the onset of an outbreak or for prevention.

DOSAGE: *one injection per week for three to four weeks until symptoms subside or monthly injections for prevention*

## Vitamin E

During an outbreak vitamin E topically may provide pain relief and promote healing. Vitamin E is also a well-known immune enhancing antioxidant when taken orally.

ORAL DOSAGE: *Take 400 IU of mixed tocopherols daily.*
*Topically during an outbreak: Apply vitamin E oil to the lesion with a Q-tip.*

## Lemon Balm – *Melissa officinalis*

The concentrated extract (70:1) of lemon balm has been used extensively in Germany for oral cold sores and more products are now available in North America. Studies using the lemon balm topically have shown very impressive results.

One study reported that when a patient used lemon balm during an initial herpes infection, there was not a single recurrence. Using the topical cream increased healing time of the lesions as well as prevented more cold sores from developing.

DOSAGE: *Apply topically two to four times a day for 7 to 10 days for increased healing and prevention of further outbreaks.*

## Licorice Root – *Glycyrrhiza glabra*

Another popular treatment for herpes outbreaks and inhibiting the HSV replication is a component found in licorice root called glycyrrhetinic acid. This compound, when applied to lesions topically, has been shown in clinical studies to be very effective in reducing the healing time and pain associated with cold sores and genital herpes.

Licorice root can also be taken orally to support immune function and to help defend against viral infections. **NOTE: Individuals who suffer from high blood pressure should not take Licorice extract orally.**

DOSAGE: *Apply ointment or gel topically two to four times daily to inactivate the virus.*

### St. John's Wort – *Hypericum perforatum*
Studies have demonstrated the strong antiviral activity of St. John's wort by its two constituents, hypericin and pseudohypericin.

DOSAGE: *Take 500 mg standardized extract twice daily on an empty stomach.*

### Bee Propolis
Bees create propolis, a natural resin, to build their hives. Historically, bee propolis has been used for various health conditions. Studies suggest that because propolis has antiviral properties it may be useful topically for HSV outbreaks.

DOSAGE: *Apply 3% bee propolis ointment four to six times per day for 10 days.*

### Aloe Vera
The transparent gel from the cactus plant, Aloe vera has been used topically for thousands of years to treat wounds, skin infections, burns and many other skin conditions. Evidence from human studies suggest that extract from Aloe vera in a cream may be an effective treatment of genital herpes in men to shorten healing time and decrease symptoms.

DOSAGE: *Apply 0.5% cream topically two to four times daily.*

## CONVENTIONAL TREATMENT

<u>Antivirals</u>

The goal of conventional antiviral medication is to limit the severity of the infection and to reduce recurrent infections.

The three medications that are most commonly prescribed are:

- Acyclovir (Zovirax)
- Valacyclovir (Valtrex)
- Famciclovir (Famvir).

---------------- CHAPTER 10 ----------------

# HEART DISEASE AND STROKE

According to the World Health Organization (WHO), it is estimated that 30% of all deaths that occur around the globe each year are from cardiovascular disease. That figure represents approximately 18 million people.

Stroke is the third-leading cause of death in Canada and each year, more than 50,000 people have strokes. Almost 300,000 Canadians are currently living with the long-term effects of stroke.

In January 2010, the Heart and Stroke Foundation designated young adults as the newest at-risk group for heart disease in Canada.

In the span of a decade, rates of high blood pressure among Canadians have jumped by 77%, diabetes by 45% and obesity by 18%. These conditions are all risks for heart disease and are becoming more prevalent among young adults. There are more than 250,000 Canadians between 20 and 30 years of age who have high blood pressure. In the age group 35 to 49, high blood pressure has increased by 127%, diabetes by 64% and obesity by 20%. This is very ALARMING!

## The Truth about Cholesterol

Cholesterol has gotten a bad reputation over the years and while it's true that too much of certain fats can cause major damage in the body, other forms are absolutely vital to our health and well-being.

Most people and some doctors still believe that excess cholesterol in the blood can lead to angina, heart attacks and strokes. But what is unreported is that not all cholesterol is harmful. In fact, you can't live without it. Cholesterol is an essential component of our cell membranes, acts as an antioxidant and a precursor for the synthesis of vitamins D, E and K. It is also a precursor for the production of steroid hormones such as cortisol and other adrenal hormones, estrogen, progesterone and testosterone and a precursor for calcitriol which regulates calcium. Cholesterol is used in brain/nerve communication and it repairs lesions in the membranes of arteries and veins.

There are two types of cholesterol: low-density lipoprotein (LDL) or "BAD" cholesterol and high-density lipoprotein (HDL) or "GOOD" cholesterol. When LDL levels get too high, plaque will slowly build up on the walls of blood vessels, narrowing the arteries and therefore, putting more stress on the heart to work harder. If too much plaque accumulates, blood flow and oxygen to the heart is obstructed, causing chest pain. If a blood clot forms and blocks the artery, a heart attack may occur.

HDL removes LDL cholesterol, carrying it back to the liver and protecting against hardening of the arteries. HDL also helps break down cholesterol into fatty acids essential for cell membrane integrity. Keeping the correct balance of LDL to HDL is essential to heart health.

## The ROOT CAUSE – CHRONIC INFLAMMATION

It is not the cholesterol levels or the cholesterol-containing foods that are the culprits in heart disease. Cholesterol has been blamed because upon inspection of the arteries of someone who has had, or is at risk for heart attack, levels of plaque containing cholesterol are very high.

Inflammation in the body can be caused by ongoing stress, poor dietary habits and a deficiency of antioxidants, to name a few. The inflammation causes damage to the lining of the blood vessels and cholesterol is transported to the tissues as part of the inflammatory response to repair the damage. It will only lodge itself onto the artery and cause plaque build up if the artery has become damaged. Cholesterol is not "the bad guy". It is becoming a well-known fact that the main cause of coronary artery disease is chronic inflammation.

Atherosclerosis is characterized by chronic inflammation involving immune system response. So, a more important question to ask is how do we prevent and decrease the amount of inflammation in our bodies, rather than how can we reduce cholesterol-containing foods and cholesterol levels?

## The Effects of STRESS

Adrenal stress hormones, called glucocorticoids are powerful anti-inflammatory agents. But in chronic stress, a problem can occur and as a result, the fight or flight response remains active. Eventually this causes cells in the immune system to release cytokines - molecules that promote inflammation.

It is clear that stress can create significant damage to the cardiovascular system by increasing the risk of coronary artery disease, elevating blood pressure, increasing atherosclerosis and increasing the risk of a heart attack.

Stress also causes the blood to become thicker. The combination of a narrowing of the arteries due to plaque and blood sludge, put considerable stress on the heart and blood vessels. Due to the narrowing of arteries and blood thickening, the blood pressure increases and plaque is often dislodged and travels in the blood stream and becomes a "ticking time bomb". If the plaque gets stuck in one of the heart arteries, it triggers a heart attack. If the plaque is trapped in a blood vessel in the brain, it can cause a stroke.

## High Blood Pressure – The Silent Killer

It seems that many chronic conditions appear without any symptoms. That is certainly true for high blood pressure. While untreated high blood pressure can lead to serious health consequences (angina, fluid in the lungs, heart damage, kidney damage, stroke, loss of memory and vision), there is little indication that it's developing. This explains why it's crucial to have your blood pressure checked regularly.

High blood pressure is the result of damage to the arteries, which are crucial to transport oxygen via the blood. Damage occurs either by cholesterol and plaque build-up, trapped blood clots and the resultant tissue damage or increased workload. Over time, organs supplied by these arteries can suffer due to lack of blood flow and eventually, the heart itself can become damaged. According to the American Heart Association, 77% of those experiencing a first stroke, 69% of those experiencing a first heart attack and 74% of those with congestive heart failure have blood pressure higher than 140/90.

## Blood Pressure Guidelines

| Blood Pressure | Systolic (mm Hg) | Diastolic (mm Hg) |
|---|---|---|
| Normal | below 120 | below 80 |
| Prehypertension | 120-139 | 80-89 |
| Stage 1 hypertension | 140-159 | 90-99 |
| Stage 2 hypertension | 160 or higher | 100 or higher |

 **FACT – Did You Know?**

A recent study published in *The Lancet* found that if the two blood pressure readings taken on both arms differ by more than 15 mm Hg, there is an increased risk of peripheral vascular disease (PVD) - the narrowing of arteries that supply blood to the legs and feet. It is also associated with an increased risk of cerebrovascular disease which affects the blood supply to the brain.

## Risk Factors

- A family history of heart disease increases your risk of heart disease, especially if a parent developed it at an early age (before age 55 for a male relative, such as a brother or father, and before age 65 for a female relative, such as a mother or sister)
- Aging increases risk of heart disease and stroke as this increases the risk of damaged and narrowed arteries and weakened or thickened heart muscle, which will contribute to heart disease
- Obesity triples the risk: waist to hip ratio is greater than 0.8 (waist

measurement divided by hip measurement) and body mass index greater than 29 (weight in kilograms divided by the square of height in metres)

- High blood pressure can result in hardening and thickening of arteries, narrowing the vessels through which blood flows.
- Smoking will increase risk 3 to 5 times
- Excessive alcohol (more than two drinks daily)
- Lack of exercise
- Increased stress
- High blood cholesterol levels, especially high LDL ("bad" cholesterol) and low HDL ("good" cholesterol), and high triglycerides
- High blood sugar, high insulin, metabolic syndrome and diabetes increases risk 3 to 7 times
- Iron excess
- Underactive thyroid
- Hormone Replacement Therapy
- Current use of birth control pill
- Postmenopausal women with lower estrogen and progesterone
- Heavy metal toxicity – especially cadmium, lead and mercury
- Excess free radicals from BBQ meat, chemicals, x-rays, UV light
- Poor diet – excess consumption of sugar, sweets and high glycemic carbohydrates, animal fats, smoked meats, fried foods, rancid oils, margarine, processed foods
- Low dietary fibre

## TESTS and DIAGNOSIS

Physical and lab tests are useful in assessing heart disease and stroke risk. This may include checking blood pressure during an annual physical exam or if there is a history of elevated blood pressure, monthly checks may be performed until it is brought under control.

My recommendation is to always keep track of your blood pressure at least every few months either at home (using a home blood pressure monitor) or at the drug store, especially if you have some of the above risk factors.

Blood tests may include:

- Total cholesterol, HDL, LDL, cholesterol/HDL ratio, LDL/HDL ratio, triglycerides

As mentioned previously, LDL cholesterol is "The Bad Guy" that transports cholesterol and triglycerides from the liver to the peripheral tissues. The high-density lipoprotein (HDL) exhibits protective effects by transporting the free cholesterol back to the liver. It is important to maintain a higher level of HDL compared to LDL. Elevated triglycerides are an important risk factor in insulin resistance as a risk for heart disease.

- Lipoprotein-a is a strong risk factor for coronary artery disease, cerebrovascular disease, atherosclerosis, thrombosis and stroke. Lipoprotein-a levels are only slightly affected by diet, exercise and other environmental factors and commonly prescribed lipid-reducing drugs have little or no effect. High Lp(a) predicts risk of early atherosclerosis similar to LDL but in advanced atherosclerosis Lp(a), it is an independent risk factor, not dependent on LDL. In cases of elevated lipoprotein-a, Aspirin has been shown to lower levels up to 80%.
- Apolipoprotein B (apoB) is the primary apolipoprotein of the low- density lipoproteins (LDL or bad cholesterol) and is responsible for carrying cholesterol to the tissues. High levels of apoB can lead to plaque that cause vascular disease (atherosclerosis) and has been found to be a better predictor of heart disease than LDL.
- C-Reactive Protein (CRP) is a general marker for infection and inflammation. Ask for the high-sensitivity CRP (hs-CRP) test.
- Homocysteine is a common amino acid and is related to early development of heart and blood vessel disease. In fact, it is considered an independent risk factor for heart disease.
- Ferritin can be a marker for inflammation and predictor for heart disease.

- Fibrinogen is a marker for blood clotting and high levels can increase risk of a heart attack or stroke.
- Heavy metal testing – Heavy metals such as cadmium, alumimum, lead and mercury can cause damage to blood vessels and increase inflammation. IV chelation may be recommended to help remove high levels of heavy metals in the body. Seek IV chelation treatments or heavy metal testing from a trained Naturopathic Doctor or Complementary Medical Doctor.
- Fasting blood sugar and insulin to assess risk of diabetes and metabolic syndrome.
- Oxidata test for free radical burden, which can lead to chronic inflammation and risk of cardiovascular disease. This test is usually performed by a Naturopathic Doctor.
- Koenisberg test for adrenal function testing (helps determine how well your body is coping with stress). This test is usually performed by a Naturopathic Doctor.

> **FACT – Did You Know?**
> Stress and the emotions associated with stress are important risk factors for cardiovascular disease. The Mayo Clinic reported the strongest risk factor among individuals with existing coronary artery disease is psychological health as a predictor of future cardiac events. When researchers interview heart attack survivors, they found the intensity and timing of stressful emotions like anger, anxiety and worry dramatically increased their risk.

For those who are symptomatic, for example with chest pain, shortness of breath or pain, numbness, weakness or coldness in legs or arms, other cardiovascular risk screening is recommended including:

- Stress test
- Holter monitoring
- Chest x-ray
- Electrocardiogram (ECG)
- Echocardiogram

- CT scan
- MRI
- IMT – carotid intima-media thickness (determines the thickness of the inside of the carotid arteries as well as the flow of blood through the arteries).

## *PREVENTION and TREATMENT – Dietary and Lifestyle*

### FOOD FACTORS

Focusing on healthy dietary habits is a foundation for keeping the heart healthy and preventing heart disease and stroke.

There has been a great deal of information in the news about lowering the amount of dietary fat to prevent heart disease. It is important to distinguish the difference between the types of fats - "good" vs "bad".

Harmful fats should be eliminated or minimized, which include saturated fats from red meat, cheese, butter, milk and, to a lesser degree, poultry.

Saturated fats are solid at room temperature and can contribute to high LDL levels ("bad" cholesterol). These should be eaten in scarce amounts to protect the heart. Unsaturated fats are liquid at room temperature and include most vegetable oils such as olive oil.

**FACT – Did You Know?**

A daily 25 ml dose of olive oil has been shown to reduce cardiovascular risk factors by increasing HDL ("good" cholesterol) levels, decreasing oxidative damage on fats and improving glutathione levels that help protect the heart against oxidative stress.

Adding hydrogen to vegetable oil through a process called "hydrogenation" makes trans fats. Commercially-baked foods (crackers, cookies, cakes) and many fried foods such as donuts and french fries, often contain trans fats. Many food manufacturers use trans fats to help foods stay fresh longer and improve shelf life.

These fats promote inflammation and increase free radicals, which damage blood vessels and increase plaque formation. They also cause elevations of insulin, cholesterol, triglycerides, LDL and lipoprotein-a. HDL ("good" cholesterol) levels are often lowered as a result.

Studies have found a strong correlation between low levels of omega-3 fatty acids and heart disease. Omega-3 fatty acids lower levels of LDL cholesterol and triglycerides, lower blood pressure in those individuals with high blood pressure and inhibit platelet aggregation. Be sure to include omega-3s in the form of fish or flax oil to help inhibit inflammation in the body thus preventing cardiovascular problems.

Other beneficial fats include those from nuts (almonds, brazil, walnuts, pecans), seeds, algae, avocado, coconut and olive oil.

Consuming adequate amounts of fibre is another important dietary habit to acquire for preventing heart disease. Fibre helps bind cholesterol and other potential toxins, promoting better elimination and preventing free radical damage to the arteries. Research has shown that when a high fibre diet is initiated, there is a reduction in a variety of cardiovascular risk factors such as hypertension, homocysteine and obesity. Excellent fibre sources include psyllium, ground flax seeds, hemp/chia seeds, legumes, oat bran and fruits and vegetables. A minimum of 40 grams of fibre should be consumed daily (see **Appendix**).

High glycemic carbohydrates (corn, white rice, millet, potatoes, boxed cereals, baked goods) are converted into glucose very quickly after being consumed and digested. An increase in glucose will raise blood sugars and send a signal to the pancreas to make insulin to help clear the glucose from the blood. The increase in insulin triggers the liver to make excess cholesterol, which can cause damage to organs and promote atherosclerosis (hardening of arteries). High glycemic and refined foods also increase triglycerides, LDL cholesterol and blood pressure.

In contrast, complex carbohydrates are high in fibre and nutrient content and are converted into glucose slowly in the body, stabilizing blood sugar and insulin levels. Brown rice, quinoa, oats, barley, whole fruits and vegetables are the preferred choice of carbohydrates for preventing heart disease.

Be sure to check labels carefully for added sugars. Foods that contain sucrose, glucose, maltose, lactose, fructose, sugar and corn syrup should be consumed as little as possible or not at all.

Inflammation is one of the main culprits in cardiovascular disease. Inflammatory foods (animal protein, dairy products, caffeine, alcohol, refined/processed foods, vegetables from the night shade family - tomatoes, peppers, eggplant, potatoes) should be eaten in moderation. Foods that will help decrease inflammation and fund antioxidants should be included in the diet (onion, garlic, ginger, green tea, turmeric, almonds, walnuts, broccoli, kale, legumes).

 **FACT – Did You Know?**

A meta-analysis of 28 controlled trials found that consuming more organic fermented soy products rather than animal protein, significantly decreased serum concentrations of total cholesterol, LDL ("bad") cholesterol and triglycerides and increased HDL ("good") cholesterol.

## LIFESTYLE TIPS

- Stay hydrated with plenty of water. A minimum of 1.5 to 2 litres should be consumed daily to help reduce cholesterol levels, improve alkalinity, remove toxins in the body, and help flush out excess sodium thus improving blood pressure.
- Keep tabs on your blood pressure. Do BP checks at least every few months if you have had high blood pressure in the past or once every six to eight months if your blood pressure is normal.
- Reduce your intake of table salt or packaged foods that contain high amounts of sodium. Choose herbs and spices to season your meals or use Celtic sea salt in moderation.
- Limit caffeine, alcohol and sugar consumption as these have all been linked to increased risk of heart disease.
- Eat more potassium-rich foods like carrot juice, grapefruit juice, banana, kiwi, potato, yam, squash and avocado.
- Don't smoke!
- Exercise a minimum of 30 to 40 minutes, three times weekly combining both aerobic and non-aerobic exercise.

- Achieve and maintain a healthy weight to reduce strain on your heart.
- Start your day with fibre-filled cereals which are cardio-protective. Include a source of protein such as nuts and enjoy it with some organic plain yogurt. This will help to ensure your blood sugar is stabilized early in the day.
- Manage stress levels – take time each day to relax, meditate, and laugh!
- Assess thyroid function as high cholesterol can be linked to an underactive thyroid function.
- Check heavy metals. Consult with an MD or ND about intravenous chelation to help with the removal of atherosclerotic plaque.
- Identify food allergies – dairy, egg, gluten, corn, peanuts or soy.

## KEY SUPPLEMENTS

### Flaxseed Oil and/or Pure Fish Oil
Essential fatty acids in the form of flaxseed or uncontaminated fish oil decrease the formation of PGE2, which is a messenger molecule that promotes inflammatory pathways in the body. Increased inflammation is associated with an increase in insult to the arteries thus promoting atherosclerosis and plaque formation. Fish oil also helps to lower triglyceride levels.

DOSAGE: *Take up to 2 Tbsp of flax oil daily and/or up to 3000 mg fish oil daily with a minimum of 1000 EPA and 600 mg DHA.*

### CoQ10
Coenzyme Q10 (ubiquinone, CoQ10) is an important antioxidant and is necessary for the health of all human tissues and organs. It is required for the production of ATP, our body's energy source.

**Body/Mind Connection**
Your heart represents the centre of love and your security. Heart problems signify long-term emotional issues. Allow joy and happiness into your life!

The use of CoQ10 for cardiovascular disease prevention and treatment is impressive. CoQ10 increases energy production in the heart muscle cells. Supplementation will improve contractility of the cardiac muscle, increase antioxidant activity within the cardiovascular system, lower blood pressure and improve heart muscle performance.

DOSAGE: *100–300 mg daily*

 **FACT – Did You Know?**

Statin (cholesterol-lowering) medications such as Lipitor or Crestor will deplete CoQ10 inside the heart muscle by inhibiting an enzyme responsible for the production of cholesterol as well as CoQ10. Many blood pressure medications will also deplete CoQ10 levels in the body. Taking CoQ10 supplements is CRITICAL for those individuals who are prescribed statin or blood pressure medications.

### *Sytrinol®*

New research shows the value in supplementing with a combination of powerful natural antioxidants including polymethoxylated flavones (PMFs) and a range of palm (alpha, delta and gamma) tocotrienols (analogues of vitamin E) to help lower total cholesterol, LDL cholesterol and triglycerides while boosting levels of the healthy HDL cholesterol.

Sytrinol® is also a powerful antioxidant with numerous heart health benefits - the reduction of arterial plaque, improved glycemic control and reduced blood platelet aggregation.

The polymethoxylated flavones, including nobiletin and tangeretin, have been found to help lower LDL cholesterol by inhibiting apolipoprotein B and triglycerides. Apolipoprotein B is considered a primary building block of the LDL cholesterol complex and triglycerides are one of the key contributors to the formation of apolipoprotein B. In addition, PMFs have been studied for their anti-inflammatory properties, which help decrease C-reactive protein (an important heart disease and inflammatory marker).

The tocotrienols (vitamin E analogues) work by controlling the degradation rate of the HMG-CoA reductase enzyme. HMG-CoA reductase is required for cholesterol synthesis in the liver and the tocotrienols help increase the rate of natural degradation of this enzyme thus reducing total cholesterol.

Studies show that the combination of the above ingredients, found in the proprietary product Sytrinol®, works independently of diet. This is great news if you are just starting to evolve your diet toward a more heart-healthy way of eating!

DOSAGE: *1 capsule daily*

## Plant Sterols – *ImmunoCare*™

Sterols interfere with the absorption of cholesterol, which is why they prove to be so beneficial in reducing high cholesterol and LDL levels. The National Institutes of Health (NIH) recommends the consumption of 1.3 grams of plant sterols daily to promote healthy cholesterol levels.

DOSAGE: *1500 mg daily*

## Niacin

Niacin has been a well-researched and established therapy in cardiovascular disease due to its ability to lower cholesterol, lower LDL and triglycerides and increase HDL cholesterol. Side effects commonly occur with niacin and many individuals will discontinue therapy due to skin "flushing" and itching. People may also experience an increase in blood glucose or uric acid levels, gastrointestinal distress, activation of peptic ulcer and liver toxicity. Inositol hexaniacinate is the form of niacin that is well tolerated. It does not cause the "flushing" or to any great extent, the side effects commonly associated with high doses of regular niacin.

DOSAGE: *500 mg one to three times daily (inositol hexaniacinate) or to avoid many of the above side effects often experienced with regular niacin begin at a lower dose of 100 mg two times daily (niacin) and titrate up gradually.*

## Vitamin E – Mixed Tocopherols

Vitamin E is known for its antioxidant, immune-enhancing, anti-inflammatory and anti-platelet aggregation effects. Many studies have shown its use in the prevention of cardiovascular disease, cancer, cataracts and complications of diabetes.

DOSAGE: *400–1000 IU daily*
*\*Note: Do not take with prescription blood thinners such as Warfarin or Coumadin.*

## Vitamin C

Vitamin C is a powerful antioxidant that helps protect the body from unstable molecules (free radicals) that eventually degenerate our healthy cells. It helps to reduce the formation of bad cholesterol and hardening of the arteries, thus preventing heart disease. Research has found that individuals with high blood pressure have accompanying low serum levels of vitamin C. Smokers will also benefit from taking this vitamin as nicotine is known for reducing blood vitamin C levels.

DOSAGE: *1000–3000 mg daily or to bowel tolerance*

## Potassium

Potassium has a key role in nerve transmission, muscle contraction, enzyme reactions, carbohydrate synthesis and acid-base balance. A diet deficient in potassium may cause high blood pressure, stroke and heart disease. The dosage of potassium is based on each individualized case and high doses may cause nausea, vomiting and diarrhea. For this reason, many practitioners encourage the eating of potassium-rich foods such as bananas, apples, carrots, potatoes and lima beans over supplementation. High levels of potassium may be contraindicated in kidney disease or impaired kidney function. In addition, potassium should be used with caution in individuals with hypoaldosteronism and in those taking medications that can cause potassium retention (potassium-sparing diuretics, angiotensin converting enzyme (ACE) inhibitors, angiotensin II receptor blockers (ARBS), nonsteroidal anti-inflammatory drugs (NSAIDs), beta blockers, digoxin).

DOSAGE: *99–300 mg daily*

## Calcium
Calcium is well known for its role in preventing osteoporosis and supporting healthy bones and teeth. But it is also vitally important for the regulation of the contraction and relaxation of heart muscle. Calcium has also been shown to be useful in reducing cholesterol and high blood pressure.

DOSAGE: *500–1200 mg daily from the diet or from supplementation as calcium citrate, malate or fumarate.*

## Magnesium Bisglycinate or citrate
Magnesium is one of the most important vitamins for cardiovascular disease prevention and heart health. It is responsible for keeping the heart strong by supporting contraction, increasing HDL levels and inhibiting platelet aggregation. Studies have shown that magnesium is beneficial for high blood pressure, arrhythmias, heart palpitations and many other heart conditions and symptoms.

DOSAGE: *400–800 mg daily*

## Vitamin D
Most people suffering from atherosclerosis and heart disease are chronically deficient in Vitamin D. There is a strong inverse relationship between vitamin D levels and artery calcification, i.e. the more vitamin in the blood, the less calcification. Artery cells have vitamin D receptors (VDR) which, when stimulated by vitamin D, inhibit the deposit of calcium.

DOSAGE: *1000–4000 IU daily*

## L-Arginine

L-arginine is an amino acid that is not only made in the body but is present in the diet as well. It is an important building block for protein synthesis and is a precursor to nitric oxide, which promotes vasodilation and relaxation of blood vessels. For this reason, L-arginine improves blood flow, reduces blood pressure and helps ease the pain from angina. L-arginine also supports the immune system and helps wound healing.

DOSAGE: *1000–3000 mg daily*

## L-Carnitine

L-carnitine is an amino acid found naturally in the body. It is synthesized in the liver, kidney and brain from lysine by a process that requires vitamin C, iron, vitamin B6 and niacin. L-carnitine plays a key role in energy production and enhances fat metabolism, thus helping to reduce total and LDL cholesterol levels and triglycerides. Individuals who take L-carnitine have demonstrated lower levels of lipoprotein-a (a marker for heart disease).

DOSAGE: *1000–3000 mg daily*

## Folic acid, B6 and B12

Homocysteine is an amino acid that our bodies produce as a by-product of tissue and muscle repair using the protein methionine. With adequate vitamin B12, folic acid and vitamin B6, our bodies can recycle homocysteine back to methionine or change it to a helpful cysteine. Without sufficient B12, folic acid, and vitamin B6 however, homocysteine levels rise, leading to increased risk of coronary heart disease, stroke and peripheral vascular disease. Elevated homocysteine has also been linked to aging, cigarette smoking and drinking too much coffee.

*Dosages: Folic acid 400 mcg–3 mg daily, Vitamin B12 400–1000 mcg daily and Vitamin B6 25–100 mg daily.*

## Hawthorn – *Crataegus oxyacantha*

The berries, leaves and flowers of Hawthorn have been used traditionally as cardiac tonics in a variety of heart disorders. The cardioprotective ingredient comes from its flavonoid content, specifically the proanthocyanidin, which gives the herb significant antioxidant activity. Hawthorn increases coronary blood flow, thus improving the utilization of oxygen by the heart. In addition, this herb is effective for hypertension, reducing cholesterol (LDL and triglycerides) and for preventing atherosclerosis and heart disease.

DOSAGE: *100–250 mg daily (1.8% vitexin or 20% procyanidins)*

## Red Yeast Rice Extract

Red yeast rice is a fermented rice produced by growing red yeast (*Monascus purpureus*) on white rice. It has been used in Asia for more than 1000 years and is a dietary staple in China and Japan. Red yeast rice extract has been observed to decrease cholesterol levels because it contains a compound called monacolin. This compound is structurally very similar to the statin drugs simvastatin, lovastatin and pravastatin. Like these drugs, the monacolins in the red yeast rice extract inhibit cholesterol synthesis by inhibiting HMG-CoA reductase, the enzyme responsible for the synthesis of cholesterol in the body.

DOSAGE: *2.4 grams daily*

## Garlic

Garlic is a popular lipid-lowering agent since it has been reported to inhibit cholesterol synthesis. It improves circulation and reduces high blood pressure. Use liberally in foods or take as a supplement.
DOSAGE: *1000–3000 mg daily*

## Thyroid Support – *ThyroSense®*

Hypothyroidism is associated with elevated levels of cholesterol. Check thyroid hormones and supplement if TSH levels are above 2.0

DOSAGE: *2 capsules twice daily*

## Adrenal Support – *AdrenaSense®*

Chronic stress promotes the release of cytokines, which are inflammatory molecules. Chronic inflammation can damage blood vessels and lead to atherosclerosis thus increasing blood pressure and the risk of heart attack and coronary heart disease.

DOSAGE: *1 capsule one to three times daily*
*Note: Siberian ginseng in AdrenaSense® is an adaptogenic herb that helps to regulate blood pressure as opposed to Panax ginseng that has been known to elevate blood pressure in some individuals. If you have high blood pressure, start with 1 capsule of AdrenaSense® a day and work up slowly while monitoring your blood pressure.*

## CONVENTIONAL MEDICINE

There are a wide variety of medications prescribed to help lower cholesterol and control high blood pressure. Unfortunately, many of these medications have unwanted side effects and deplete important vitamins and minerals. Talk to your Naturopathic Doctor or complementary health care practitioner to ensure that you are taking the appropriate vitamins and minerals if you have been prescribed any of the following medications:

### Water Pills – Diuretics

Diuretics help get rid of excess water and salt through the urine, which lessens the burden on the heart and lowers high blood pressure. Examples include:

- Lasix (furosemide)
- Esidrix (hydrochlorothiazide)
- Aldactone (spironolactone)
- Demadex (torsemide)
- Zaroxolyn (metolazone).

Loop diuretics such as furosemide cause nutrient depletions of zinc, sodium, calcium, magnesium, potassium and vitamins B1, B6 and C.

Thiazide diuretics such as hydrochlorothiazide cause nutrient depletions of magnesium, potassium, zinc, CoQ10 and sodium.

Potassium-sparing diuretics such as spironolactone deplete calcium, folic acid and zinc.

Medical doctors often prescribe diuretics if you have:

- Edema/swelling in the legs
- High blood pressure
- Heart Failure
- Liver problems.

## ACE Inhibitors – Angiotensin converting enzyme (ACE) inhibitors

ACE inhibitors help widen or dilate blood vessels to improve the amount of blood the heart pumps and help lower high blood pressure. ACE inhibitors also increase blood flow which means that your heart does not have to work as hard.

Examples include:

- Altace (ramipril)
- Vasotec (enalapril)
- Accupril (quinapril)
- Capoten (captopril).

ACE inhibitors deplete sodium and zinc and are often prescribed if you have:

- High blood pressure
- Heart failure
- History of heart attack
- Diabetes
- Heart disease.

Beta-Blockers
Beta-blockers improve the heart's ability to relax, decrease the production of harmful substances produced by the body in response to heart failure and slow the heart rate. Over time, they can improve the heart's pumping ability.
Examples include:

- Coreg (carvedilol)
- Lopressor (metoprolol)
- Tenormin (atenolol)
- Inderal (propranolol)
- Zebeta (bisoprolol)
- Sectral (acebutolol).

Beta-blockers deplete CoQ10 and melatonin and are often prescribed if you have:

- High blood pressure
- Heart failure
- Angina
- Abnormal heart rhythms
- Have had a heart attack.

Sometimes beta-blockers are prescribed for glaucoma, migraine headaches and performance anxiety.

Calcium Channel Blockers
Calcium channel blockers relax blood vessels and increase the supply of blood and oxygen to the heart, reducing the heart's workload.
Examples include:

- Norvasc (amlodipine)
- Plendil (felodipine)
- Cardizem/Tiazac (diltiazem)

- Calan (verapamil)
- Adalat (nifedipine).

Calcium channel blockers deplete potassium and are often prescribed if you have:

- Coronary artery disease/Coronary spasm
- Angina
- Abnormal heart rhythms
- Hypertrophic cardiomyopathy.

## ARBs – Angiotensin II Receptor Blockers

ARBs work similarly to ACE inhibitors but by a different mechanism. Since they decrease certain chemicals that narrow blood vessels, blood is allowed to flow more easily through the body. ARBs also decrease chemicals that cause salt and fluid build-up in the body.
Examples include:

- Cozaar (losartan)
- Diovan (valsartan)
- Avapro (irbesartan)
- Atacand (candesartan)
- Micardis (telmisartan).

ARBs are often prescribed if you cannot tolerate an ACE inhibitor.

## Cardiac Glycosides – Digoxin

Digoxin helps an injured or weakened heart work more efficiently to send blood through the body. It strengthens the force of the heart muscle's contractions, slows the heart rate and improves blood circulation.

Digoxin depletes vitamin B1, calcium, magnesium and phosphorus. It is often prescribed to treat:

- Heart failure
- Atrial fibrillation.

## Cholesterol-lowering Medications – Statins

Statins block the production of cholesterol in the liver by blocking the enzyme HMG-CoA reductase which is responsible for cholesterol synthesis.

Examples include:

- Atorvastatin (Lipitor)
- Fluvastatin (Lescol)
- Lovastatin (Mevacor)
- Pravastatin (Pravachol)
- Simvastatin (Zocor)
- Rosuvastatin (Crestor).

Statins deplete CoQ10.

Other conventional medications often prescribed for prevention or treatment of cardiovascular disease include:

- Aspirin
- Coumadin/Warfarin.

—————————— CHAPTER 11 ——————————

# HYPOTHYROIDISM

## A Little on Thyroid Health...

It is estimated that 200 million people in the world have some form of thyroid disease. In Canada there is a staggering number of people affected with this condition. Recent studies indicate that one in every three Canadians has a thyroid disorder. Of those, as many as 50% are undiagnosed!

The thyroid gland is a small, butterfly-shaped gland located in the base of the neck on both sides of the lower part of the voice box (larynx) and upper part of the wind pipe (trachea). The thyroid produces hormones called thyroxine (T4) and triiodothyronine (T3), which regulate the body's metabolism by controlling body temperature, the synthesis of protein and the release of energy from the cells.

Thyroxine (T4) is the most abundant thyroid hormone produced (about 93%) and at one time was thought to be the active hormone. However, we now know that triiodothyronine (T3) is three to five times more active biologically and it is the active hormone in target cells.

T4 is converted to T3 in the liver, kidneys and body cells (about 80%) and the thyroid is responsible for the rest. When blood levels of T3 and T4 increase, the pituitary gland slows production of TSH.

## The Role of the THYROID GLAND

The thyroid's job is to increase the body's metabolic rate by increasing the activity of the mitochondria (the body's energy producers). The mitochondria use oxygen to convert energy from food into carbon dioxide, water, heat and energy for the body. Thyroid hormones are responsible for maintaining body temperature, stimulating protein synthesis, increasing the use of glucose and the breakdown of fats for energy production. They speed up the elimination of cholesterol into bile from the liver. Thyroid hormones affect mood, emotions, memory and the way we think by increasing the growth of nervous tissue.

## Hypothyroidism

Hypothyroidism (underactive or low thyroid function) occurs when the thyroid gland fails to produce sufficient amounts of the thyroid hormones T4 and T3 or there is a failure in the conversion of T4 to T3. It is more common in females, affecting 20 to 25% of the female population in North America and about 10% of males.

## SIGNS and SYMPTOMS

The signs and symptoms of hypothyroidism vary widely, depending on the severity of the hormone deficiency. But in general, any problems that arise tend to develop slowly, often over a number of years.

Some of the common signs and symptoms of hypothyroidism include:

- Fatigue, muscle weakness, lethargy
- Cold intolerance, cold hands and feet, difficulty staying warm, low body temperature (underarm temperature lower than 37 C)
- Low blood pressure, high cholesterol, slow pulse, sleep apnea
- Hair loss, dry, brittle coarse hair, loss of lateral one-third of eyebrow
- Dry, pale, scaly skin, tendency to eczema, psoriasis
- Thin, brittle nails with transverse grooves
- Yellow or orange discoloration of skin – especially on the palms
- Constipation

- Headaches
- Depression, memory loss, poor concentration
- Low libido
- Puffy face, especially around the eyes, swelling of hands and feet
- Weight gain, difficulty losing weight
- Frequent or chronic infections
- Muscle aches and swelling in joints (fibromyalgia, rheumatoid arthritis, tendonitis)
- Hormonal imbalances (heavier than normal menstrual periods, PMS, endometriosis, PCOS, fibroids, ovarian cysts or severe menopausal symptoms)
- Hoarse voice
- Goiter
- Infertility, miscarriage.

Other conditions associated with hypothyroidism:
- Arthritis
- Adrenal fatigue
- Anemia
- Cardiac disease
- Depression
- Diabetes
- Lupus
- Osteoporosis
- Reproductive issues
- Psoriasis/Urticaria (itchy skin)
- Allergic rhinitis.

Advanced hypothyroidism, known as myxedema, is rare, but when it does occur, it can be life threatening. Signs and symptoms include low blood pressure, decreased breathing, decreased body temperature, unresponsiveness and even coma.

## Hypothyroidism in CHILDREN and TEENS

Although hypothyroidism most often affects middle-aged and older women, anyone can develop the condition, including infants and teenagers. Initially, babies born without a thyroid gland or with a gland that doesn't work properly may have few signs and symptoms. When newborns do have problems with hypothyroidism, they may include:

- Yellowing of the skin and whites of the eyes (jaundice). In most cases, this occurs when a baby's liver can't metabolize a substance called bilirubin, which normally forms when the body recycles old or damaged red blood cells
- Frequent choking
- A large, protruding tongue
- A puffy appearance to the face.

As the disease progresses, infants are likely to have trouble feeding and may fail to grow and develop normally. They may also have:

- Constipation
- Poor muscle tone
- Excessive sleepiness.

When hypothyroidism in infants isn't treated, even mild cases can lead to severe physical and mental developmental problems.

In general, children and teens that develop hypothyroidism have the same signs and symptoms as adults do, but they may also experience:

- Poor growth, resulting in short stature
- Delayed development of permanent teeth
- Delayed puberty
- Poor mental development.

## CAUSES

When the thyroid gland fails to produce enough of the hormones T4 and T3, the balance of chemical reactions in your body can be disrupted.

Hypothyroidism may be due to a number of different factors, including:

- *Autoimmune disease.* Hashimoto's thyroiditis is a very common cause of low thyroid. Autoimmune disorders occur when the immune system produces antibodies that attack its own tissues. In this case, the ability of the thyroid gland to produce hormones is affected and thyroid function is depressed.
- *Treatment for hyperthyroidism.* Some individuals will suffer from hyperthyroidism, where the thyroid gland will produces too much thyroid hormone. These individuals may be treated with radioactive iodine or anti-thyroid medications to reduce and normalize their thyroid function. This treatment often results in permanent hypothyroidism.
- *Radiation therapy.* Radiation used to treat cancers of the head and neck can affect the thyroid gland and may lead to hypothyroidism. Radiation exposure from x-rays, nuclear fallout, and being close to nuclear power plants can dramatically affect thyroid function.
- *Thyroid surgery.* Removing the whole thyroid or a large portion of the thyroid can reduce or stop thyroid hormone production. A majority of these cases need thyroid medication for life.
- *Medications.* There are a number of medications that can contribute to hypothyroidism. Lithium, used to treat psychiatric disorders, is one such medication. Lithium will inhibit thyroid hormone secretion. Other medications such as phenobarbitol, benzodiazepines, calcium channel blockers and steroids can increase the metabolism of thyroid hormones so that they are used up faster.
- *Heavy Metals.* Lead, mercury and cadmium can interfere with the liver's conversion of T4 to T3. High levels of mercury are often due to mercury dental fillings or consumption of high amounts of fish, particularly tuna.
- *Times of hormonal transition.* Pregnancy, menopause and childbirth can affect thyroid function as hormones are shifting quite

dramatically. Sometimes during pregnancy, women can produce antibodies against their own thyroid gland. If left untreated, hypothyroidism increases the risk of miscarriage, premature delivery and preeclampsia – a condition that causes a significant rise in blood pressure during the last three months of pregnancy. It can also seriously affect the developing fetus.

- *Stress.* The adrenal glands and thyroid gland work very closely together and during times of stress the adrenal glands are working overtime adding more stress on the thyroid and its ability to function optimally. During times of stress, excess cortisol causes diminished conversion of T4 to T3; low cortisol and adrenal fatigue may precede low thyroid disease.

- *Estrogen Dominance.* Hormone replacement therapy (synthetic or bio-identical), the birth control pill and other environmental estrogens can affect thyroid function by blocking thyroid hormone receptors.

- *Iodine Deficiency.* The mineral iodine is essential for the production of thyroid hormones.

- *Iron and other vitamin deficiencies.* Low levels of zinc, selenium, copper, magnesium, manganese, or vitamins A, B2, B3, B6, B12, C and E can cause or contribute to low thyroid function.

- *Food Allergies.* Certain foods such as gluten, dairy and animal protein can contribute to stress on the immune system as well as adrenal and thyroid function.

- *Candida.* An overgrowth of candida and bowel toxicity from food allergens can affect thyroid function.

- *Sluggish liver or liver disease.* The liver is one of the target organs that helps with the conversion of T4 to T3.

- *Pituitary disorder.* A relatively rare cause of hypothyroidism is the failure of the pituitary gland to produce enough TSH – usually because of a benign tumour of the pituitary gland.

- *Congenital disease.* Approximately 1 in 3,000 babies in the United States is born with a defective thyroid gland or no thyroid gland at all. In most cases the thyroid gland never developed normally or

some children have an inherited form of the disorder.
- *Other environmental toxins.* Perchlorate in synthetic fertilizers will inhibit the ability of the thyroid gland to trap iodine. PCBs can mimic thyroid hormone and activate an autoimmune thyroid process such as Hashimoto's.

**FACT – Did You Know?**

Most women who are approaching menopause will experience symptoms of low thyroid. Because many symptoms of thyroid imbalance are similar to menopausal symptoms, it will often go unnoticed. Don't assume that symptoms are due to peri-menopause or menopause. There could be an underlying thyroid disorder so be sure to investigate further.

## RISK FACTORS
- Female over age 50
- An autoimmune disease
- A close relative, parent or grandparent with an autoimmune disease
- Previously treated with radioactive iodine or anti-thyroid medications
- Radiation to your neck or upper chest
- History of thyroid surgery

## TESTING and DIAGNOSIS
Hypothyroidism is often more prevalent in older women, and for this reason many older women are regularly screened for low thyroid disease during routine annual physical examinations. Some doctors also recommend that pregnant women or women thinking about becoming pregnant be tested for low thyroid.

The diagnosis of hypothyroidism is based on symptoms and the results of blood tests that measure the levels of TSH, free T3, free T4, reverse T3, thyroid antimicrosomal antibodies (TPO Abs), and antithyroglobulin antibodies (Tg Abs).

Commonly, TSH is the only blood test ordered by most medical doctors and thyroid function is considered normal if the TSH falls between 0.38 to 5.5 IU/ml. However, naturopathic doctors and some medical doctors are using a new "norm" for the TSH lab value and will treat for hypothyroidism if the TSH lab value is above 1.9 especially with accompanying low thyroid symptoms. Although most medical doctors will only test TSH, it is important to measure the levels of actual thyroid hormones T4 and T3 to get a more accurate picture of the function of the thyroid. Remember that because T4 must be converted to the active form T3, tests that only measure T4 don't illustrate the whole thyroid picture. It's possible that your circulating T4 levels are in a healthy range, but you might have a problem converting T4 to T3. Be sure to ask the doctor to test levels of both hormones.

TSH alone and the old lab reference range are often inadequate and many hypothyroid patients suffer needlessly for years.

<u>Basal Body Temperature - BBT</u>
The basal body temperature is an easy way to test thyroid function and reflects metabolic rate, which is determined by the levels of thyroid hormones secreted. The basal body temperature should be taken first thing in the morning before getting out of bed. Normal basal body temperature should be between 36.6 to 36.8 degree Celsius. Normal fluctuations occur during the menstrual period (BBT will rise just after ovulation). If the BBT is consistently lower than this, low thyroid may be diagnosed. There are many other causes for low BBT and these should be ruled out before the diagnosis of hypothyroidism can be made.

Other causes for low BBT are:

- Low progesterone
- Low cortisol (adrenal fatigue)
- Low iron
- Depression
- Post-traumatic stress disorder
- Fasting
- Eating disorders

- Poor circulation
- Kidney failure.

### FACT – Did You Know?

Wilson's Temperature Syndrome is a thyroid disorder that occurs when there is a low temperature and an excess of reverse T3 (RT3) because the liver is unable to convert T4 to T3. The enzyme responsible for this conversion is dependent on selenium and zinc, vitamin B12, and the amino acid cysteine. Heavy metals such as mercury, cadmium, and lead will also block this conversion in the liver. Adrenal stress and adrenal fatigue are also culprits in Wilson's Temperature Syndrome and therefore, adrenal function should be assessed if levels of RT3 are high. Naturopathic doctors and some medical doctors usually test levels of RT3.

## *PREVENTION and TREATMENT – Dietary and Lifestyle*

### FOOD FACTORS

Nutrition should focus on supporting the health of the thyroid gland and promoting the conversion of T4 to T3.

You will recall that iodine is an essential nutrient for the production of thyroid hormones. While there are many benefits to reducing salt intake, doing so might contribute to the current epidemic of hypothyroidism. Iodized salt was a major source of dietary iodine for many North Americans - by eliminating salt, we have eliminated the source of this important nutrient for many people. If you have subclinical or clinical hypothyroidism, be sure to boost your intake of iodine-rich foods including seafood and sea vegetables (dulse, kelp, nori, hiziki, wakame). Other food sources of iodine include fish, asparagus, garlic, sea salt, sesame seeds, soybeans, spinach, summer squash and turnip greens.

Tyrosine is a building block for thyroid hormones T4 and T3. Try to include food sources of tyrosine in the diet such as sunflower seeds, pumpkin seeds, lima beans, eggs, poultry, fish, spirulina, soy and aduki beans.

Because vitamin D is a co-factor in manufacturing thyroid hormone, a deficiency in this nutrient may also be connected with hypothyroidism. Enjoy Vitamin D in shrimp, sardines, cod and eggs.

The antioxidant selenium protects the thyroid gland from stressors, and helps the body recycle its stores of iodine. Shiitake mushrooms, salmon, oats, Brazil nuts and garlic are sources of selenium. Be sure that you have plenty of B vitamins on the menu, too, as these are involved in the manufacture of T4. You'll find B Vitamins in brewer's yeast, wheat germ, sunflower seeds and legumes.

Since cold intolerance is a common symptom of hypothyroidism, use warming foods such as cinnamon, ginger, cayenne, and fennel to help thyroid imbalance.

There are many environmental toxins that can inhibit optimal thyroid function. Be sure to consume hormone and antibiotic-free meat, choose low mercury content fish and if consuming dairy, always buy organic. Many autoimmune thyroid conditions are affected by certain food allergens. If an autoimmune thyroid disease is suspected, try to avoid wheat and other gluten-containing grains as well as all dairy products.

Goitrogens are a group of foods that can interfere with the thyroid gland's ability to use iodine when dietary iodine is deficient.

Goitrogens include the brassica family of vegetables (cabbage, broccoli, Brussels sprouts, cauliflower, kale, turnips, kohlrabi, rutabaga) as well as mustard seeds, peanuts, pine nuts, millet, spinach, peaches, pears and soy.

Cooking these foods usually inactivates goitrogens and their effect is minimized if iodine-rich foods are consumed with them. It is important to note that goitrogens do not cause thyroid disease. They may only worsen an already-diagnosed hypothyroid condition.

## LIFESTYLE TIPS
- Consume high-quality protein, including antibiotic and hormone-free meats, fish, organic eggs, organic soy (in moderation), legumes, nuts and seeds.
- Eat your largest meal at breakfast and include protein with the meal.

- Eat as many fresh, organic foods as you can, while avoiding processed foods, alcohol, nicotine, coffee and caffeine. Enjoy herbal teas containing ashwagandha root, sarsaparilla root, lemongrass herb, astragalus root, ginger and peppermint leaves.
- Limit your exposure to perfluorooctanoic acid (PFOA) and perfluoroctane sulphonate (PFOS) used in various consumer products such as non-stick pans (PFOA) and stain repellants (PFOS). Research from the U.S. links these chemicals with thyroid disease.
- If you have a hypothyroid condition, determine whether you have a Candida overgrowth as the two conditions often exist together.
- Consider having mercury fillings replaced, as research shows that mercury inhibits the liver's conversion of T4 to the active thyroid hormone T3 and displaces iodine in the body. Also consider chelation therapy (the removal of heavy metals from the body) to lessen stress on the body and to improve thyroid functioning.
- Regular aerobic exercise improves blood vessel health in those with subclinical hypothyroid. Enjoy dancing, brisk walking and cycling.
- Consider doing a gentle liver detox using milk thistle, dandelion and globe artichoke. Supplement with NAC, curcumin, alpha lipoic acid, zinc, selenium, magnesium and B vitamins so that the liver is able to manage estrogen metabolism and the conversion of T4 into T3.
- Practice yoga, meditation, relaxation, deep breathing, tai chi and music or dance to help the body's adaptation to stress and restore adrenal health.
- Organochlorine pesticides (made from carbon, hydrogen and chlorine) and dioxins may reduce the lifespan of serum T4. Choose organic produce whenever possible and avoid bleached paper products (see **Breast Cancer** Chapter).

**FACT – Did You Know?**
Adrenal fatigue and hypothyroidism are often experienced at the same time because of the close relationship between adrenal and thyroid function. If thyroid disease is suspected, always treat the adrenal glands first or along with thyroid support.

## KEY SUPPLEMENTS

### L-Tyrosine
Tyrosine is an important amino acid precursor for the synthesis of thyroid hormones T4 and T3, melanin and the brain neurotransmitters dopamine, epinephrine and norepinephrine. During the stress response, the above neurotransmitters are produced by the adrenal glands. If tyrosine levels are drained, the adrenal glands cannot respond to stress adequately and there is less available to help with the synthesis of thyroid hormones.

DOSAGE: *500–1000 mg daily with food*

### Iodine
Iodine is essential for synthesis of thyroid hormones.

DOSAGE: *100–1000 mcg daily. Start with a lower dosage and increase gradually. Higher dosages are typically indicated for those individuals exposed to radiation.*
*\*\*Iodine should not be consumed in supplement form if diagnosed with hyperthyroidism (an over-active thyroid).*

### Ashwagandha - *Withania somnifera*
Ashwagandha is an important herb in Ayurvedic medicine. It serves as an adaptogen, helping the adrenal glands combat stress. As well, the herb supports healthy thyroid function by supporting the synthesis of thyroid hormones.

DOSAGE: *300–1000 mg daily*

### Guggal Extract - *Commiphora mukul*
Guggal extract has been shown to impact thyroid hormone conversion, by increasing levels of the thyroid hormone T3 peripherally in the body.

DOSAGE: *250-500 mg one to three times daily*

### Pantothenic acid - Vitamin B5
Both animal and human studies suggest that pantothenic acid is needed for adrenal function and is involved in the stress response.

Recall that adrenal function and thyroid function are closely linked. Ensuring that the adrenal glands are functioning optimally is key to supporting healthy thyroid function.

DOSAGE: *100-500 mg daily with food*

### Copper
Copper plays an important role in thyroid metabolism, especially in hormone production and absorption. Copper stimulates the production of thyroxine hormone (T4) and prevents over-absorption of T4 in the blood cells by controlling the body's calcium levels (calcium is required for the stabilization of cell membranes and reduces cell permeability).

DOSAGE: *500 mcg daily with food*

### Manganese
New scientific research is showing the vital role of manganese in liver function, fat metabolism and liver antioxidant status. This relates to thyroid hormone activation as most activation occurs on cell membranes in the liver. Manganese also serves as an antioxidant protector of the thyroid hormones. By doing so, manganese helps to support increased metabolic rate and healthy thyroid function.

DOSAGE: *500 mcg daily with food*

***All the above ingredients are found in **ThyroSense®**, an excellent product for supporting symptoms of hypothyroidism by maintaining healthy levels of T4 and T3 thyroid hormones.

DOSAGE: *Take 2 capsules with breakfast and 2 capsules with lunch.*
**ThyroSense®** *may be used with medication prescribed to increase thyroid function (e.g. Synthroid) but **NOT** in Hyperthyroid cases (over-active thyroid).*

## Bladderwrack – *Fucus vesiculosis*
Bladderwrack is brown seaweed that grows on the northern coasts of the Atlantic and Pacific oceans and the North and Baltic seas.

It contains variable levels of iodine. As a result, it has been used to treat thyroid disorders such as goiters.

DOSAGE: *200–600 mg daily*

## Selenium
A deficiency in selenium reduces the conversion of T4 into active T3 and increases the production of rT3. It is important to ensure that selenium levels are adequate for healthy thyroid function.

DOSAGE: *200-500 mcg daily*

## CONVENTIONAL MEDICINE
Calcium and iron supplements will interfere with thyroid medication or thyroid hormone supplements. Always take them at least an hour away from any thyroid supplements including medication.

The most commonly prescribed conventional medication for hypothyroidism is levothyroxine (Synthroid) which is a synthetic form of T4. In some cases, Synthroid works well but individuals who are unable to convert T4 into T3, will still experience symptoms of low thyroid while on this medication.

These individuals may respond better to Armour (desiccated thyroid extract). Some conventional doctors and naturopathic doctors may pre-scribe Armour thyroid, which is desiccated from a pig. Dosages range from 60 to 120 mg and because it contains both T4 and T3, some indi-viduals may respond to it better than synthetic Synthroid medication.

# CHAPTER 12

# INFERTILITY

Most couples achieve pregnancy within the first six months of trying to conceive. After 12 months of unprotected sexual intercourse, approximately 90% of couples will be successful. However, in Canada at the present time, almost one in six couples will have difficulty getting pregnant.

Infertility, in women under the age of 35, is defined as not being able to get pregnant despite having frequent, unprotected sexual intercourse for at least one year. For women 35 years of age or older, the time period is six months.

Studies show that 40% of the time, infertility is caused by female factors, 40% by male factors and 20% by a combination of both.

## RISK FACTORS

Common risk factors for fertility in both females and males are the same and may include:

- Age – After the age of 30, a woman's fertility gradually declines. Infertility in older women is typically due to a higher rate of chromosomal abnormalities. Men over 40 years of age may be less fertile than younger men.
- Smoking – Nicotine is toxic to the reproductive system. A couple's

chance of conceiving is reduced if either partner smokes. Miscarriages are more frequent in women who smoke.

- Alcohol – Alcohol has been linked to decreased fertility. It may be wise to eliminate it for both partners if there are fertility issues.
- Overweight – Women who are overweight are more likely to experience problems with ovulation or miscarriages. Excess abdominal fat decreases insulin sensitivity causing insulin resistance and ovulation dysfunction.
- Underweight – Women who are underweight have infrequent ovulation or may not ovulate at all.
- Exercise – Exercising more than seven hours a week has been associated with ovulation problems.
- Caffeine – Drinking coffee has been associated with decreased fertility so choose for herbal teas instead.
- Stress – Infertility issues can be very stressful and emotionally draining for both partners. Stress hormones have an inhibitory effect on the reproductive system. Therefore, addressing the stress response and adrenal function should be assessed in couples who are having fertility issues.
- Environment – Environmental toxins such as heavy metals, pesticides, and estrogen mimickers (BPA, phthalates) have been linked to many cases of infertility. These chemicals can affect sperm count, sperm formation, ovulation, hormone levels, and egg viability.

## CAUSES

Causes of female infertility include:

- Ovulation problems – eggs not being released
- Fallopian tube damage or blockage – possibly from inflammation of the tube, usually caused by Chlamydia
- Endometriosis – uterine tissue implants and grows outside the uterus often affecting sperm, egg and ovaries, uterus and fallopian tubes

- Elevated prolactin – a hormone that stimulates breast milk production, often elevated in polycystic ovarian syndrome
- Uterine fibroids – benign tumors in the wall of the uterus that may interfere with proper implantation of the fertilized egg
- General health and lifestyle – poor nutrition, obesity, use of alcohol, tobacco or drugs
- Premature ovarian failure (early menopause) – early depletion of ovarian follicles before age 40
- Elevated TSH – hypothyroidism
- Prior use of anti-estrogens (drugs such as Lupron, Depo-Provera)
- Polycystic ovarian syndrome
- Cushing's disease, kidney disease and diabetes.

Causes of male infertility include:

- Varicocele - forms when valves inside the veins along the cord that holds up a man's testicles prevent blood from flowing properly. This causes the blood to back up, leading to swelling and widening of the veins.
- Abnormal sperm production or function – due to undescended testicles, genetic defects or repeated infections
- General health and lifestyle – poor nutrition, obesity, use of alcohol, tobacco or drugs
- Overexposure to environmental factors – pesticides and other chemicals. Frequent exposure to heat, such as in saunas or hot tubs, may impair sperm production and lower sperm count
- Radiation and chemotherapy – can greatly reduce sperm count especially if treatment is to the testicles
- Age – Men over 40 may be less fertile than younger men
- Developmental abnormalities – vas deferens absence (related to cystic fibrosis), impaired testicular function (chromosome abnormality)
- Testicular surgeries or injury
- Genitourinary infection or sexually transmitted disease.

## TESTS and DIAGNOSIS

To determine the cause of infertility, a detailed medical history outlining the menstrual cycle and sexual habits as well as a physical exam may be performed (this usually includes a gynecological exam).

### Tests for Women

For a woman to be fertile, all her reproductive organs must be healthy and functional. The ovaries must release healthy eggs that are then allowed to pass into the fallopian tubes where they can be fertilized by a sperm.

Further fertility testing may include:

- Thyroid testing – Basal body temperature test, TSH, T3, T4, rT3, thyroid antibodies
- Adrenal function tests – to make sure adrenal response is healthy (see **Adrenal Fatigue** Chapter)
- Ovulation testing including hormones – estrogen, progesterone, FSH, LH, prolactin as well as charting basal body temperature.
- Pelvic ultrasound – to rule out uterine or fallopian tube disease (uterine fibroids or ovarian cysts)
- Laparoscopy – to assess possible damage to fallopian tubes, ovaries and uterus caused by endometriosis, previous ectopic pregnancy, or congenital abnormality
- Hysterosalpingography – evaluates the condition of the uterus and fallopian tubes. Fluid is injected into the uterus and then an x-ray is taken to determine if the cavity is normal and there are no blockages.
- Androgen and prolactin levels – to rule out polycystic ovarian syndrome
- Blood sugars and insulin levels – checking for diabetes and polycystic ovarian syndrome.

*Tests for Men*

For a man to be fertile, the testicles must produce enough healthy sperm and the sperm ejaculated effectively.

Further fertility testing may include:

- General physical exam – reviewing medical history, medications, any illnesses, infections (STDs) and sexual habits
- Semen analysis – to rule out motility issues, low sperm count, abnormal sperm, antibodies to sperm
- Hormone testing – to evaluate testosterone and other male hormones
- Transrectal and scrotal ultrasound – to rule out retrograde ejaculation or any duct obstructions
- Adrenal function tests – (see **Adrenal Fatigue** Chapter).

## *PREVENTION and TREATMENT – Dietary and Lifestyle*

### FOOD FACTORS

As mentioned above under risk factors, men and women should focus on daily exercise, and eat a whole foods diet free of processed and refined foods, alcohol, and caffeine. They need to avoid artificial sugars and high glycemic foods to maintain healthy blood sugar balance. The diet should consist of complex carbohydrates in the form of legumes, fruits and vegetables (stick to low glycemic – see **Appendix**), quinoa, oats and brown rice.

It is important to limit or avoid certain kinds of fish due to their mercury content since heavy metals play a role in infertility for both men and women. Prior to pregnancy, keep omega-3 fatty acids in the diet by consuming a pure, pharmaceutical grade fish oil supplement which is free of environmental toxins and mercury.

Nutritional deficiencies such as folic acid, iron, zinc, vitamin B6 and iodine can cause infertility problems. Include foods rich in these vitamins.

- Folic acid: lentils, spinach, collard greens, beans (black, garbanzo, pinto)
- Iron: soybeans, tofu, lentils, leafy vegetables (spinach), beef, prunes, garbanzo beans
- Zinc: oysters, pumpkin seeds, sesame seeds and tahini, beef and lamb, spelt
- Vitamin B6: fish, chicken, sunflower and sesame seeds, rice bran, garlic, molasses, hazelnuts
- Iodine: sea vegetables (kelp, arame, hiziki, kombu, wakame), cranberries, navy beans, yogurt, strawberries

## LIFESTYLE TIPS

- Buy organic whenever possible. Pesticides have raised some concern for fertility issues in both men and women.
- Identify food allergies and rule out celiac disease or gluten intolerance. Food allergies could lead to impaired reproductive function. Celiac disease has been associated with infertility.
- Don't smoke!
- Reduce exposure to environmental pollutants, household and industrial cleaners, solvents, heavy metals, bisphenol-A or BPA (found in plastics), and phthalates (found in beauty products). These increase the toxic burden on the body and damage eggs and sperm.
- Store food in glass, avoid canned food (most cans are lined with BPA) and do not use aluminum cookware.
- Practice stress reduction techniques. Stress can affect healthy hormone balance thus affecting fertility. Use yoga, meditation, massage, acupuncture or deep breathing exercises daily.
- Heavy metals, especially lead, mercury, aluminum, arsenic and cadmium greatly affect fertility. For this reason, you should eliminate fish from your diet that contain medium to high levels of mercury (marlin, tilefish, shark, halibut, sablefish, albacore, yellowfin tuna). If you do eat fish, consume low mercury fish and only once a week (salmon, pollock, tilapia, herring, Arctic char).
- Consider a gentle cleanse to detoxify any toxins which may have

built up in the body over time.

- Switch to drinking herbal teas such as nettle, red raspberry or red clover that will enhance fertility. Give up caffeinated beverages (e.g. coffee, black tea, sodas).
- If you have recently been on the birth control pill, address nutrient depletions (see **Birth Control** Chapter).
- Exercise at least three to five times a week combining aerobic, core strength and weight resistance. Walking, swimming, jogging, yoga, and Pilates are some excellent forms of exercise to include in an exercise routine. It may be best to limit exercise to less than seven hours a week.
- Drink at least one litre of pure filtered water daily.
- Castor oil packs, placed over the abdomen, can increase circulation and support immune function. These packs are recommended between Days 5 and 12 of a woman's cycle but should be avoided during pregnancy and menstruation. (see **Appendix** – *Castor Oil Packs*)
- Daily skin brushing (with a loofah or soft brush) removes dead skin cells. It may also improve circulation and thus assist the body in removing toxins and stimulating hormones (see **Appendix** – *Dry Skin Brushing*).

## KEY SUPPLEMENTS

### Folic Acid
Folic acid is an essential vitamin in pregnancy for the prevention of neural tube defects. Studies have shown that infertile women are deficient in this vitamin. Supplementation with folic acid has been known to reverse infertility.

DOSAGE: *1 mg daily*

### Vitamin B6
Vitamin B6 helps to normalize progesterone levels and has been shown

to be helpful for women who have premenstrual tension.

DOSAGE: *100 mg daily*

## Vitamin B12 – Methylcobalamin

Studies have shown improvements in male sperm count and improved sperm motility as well as improved fertility in women.

DOSAGE: *1000–5000 mcg daily*

## Vitamin C

Vitamin C is a powerful antioxidant that can help decrease sperm damage and may play a role in sperm motility. It is also beneficial for infertile women by improving ovarian function and in some cases, has enhanced the effect of clomiphene (a fertility drug). Vitamin C helps to increase progesterone levels and is critical for smokers.

DOSAGE: *1000–3000 mg daily or to bowel tolerance*

## Vitamin E – Mixed Tocopherols

Vitamin E helps support healthy sperm by inhibiting damage from free radicals and by increasing male fertility. Vitamin E has also been shown to be helpful for the prevention of miscarriages.

DOSAGE: *400 IU daily*

## Iron

Studies have shown that women who are iron deficient or borderline low iron may have difficulty conceiving.

DOSAGE: *15–20 mg daily*

## Selenium

Selenium is an important mineral that protects the body from free radical damage. Free radicals are unstable chemicals formed in response to environmental toxins, such as those from cigarette smoke or ingestion of excessive amounts of deep-fried and barbecued foods.

The antioxidant properties of selenium help prevent chromosomal damage and protect the body from environmental toxicity thus enhancing male and female fertility.

DOSAGE: *100–200 mcg daily*

## Zinc
Zinc is important for sperm development, count and motility. Zinc deficiency is associated with a higher incidence of miscarriages and chromosomal abnormalities. It also protects against heavy metal toxicity.

DOSAGE: *30 mg daily*

*\*Note: Many of the above vitamins and minerals can be found in a good quality prenatal multivitamin.*

## Flaxseed Oil and/or Pure Fish Oil
Essential fatty acids in the form of flaxseed or uncontaminated fish oil decrease the formation of PGE2, a type of prostaglandin that acts as a messenger molecule to promote inflammatory pathways in the body. Prostaglandins are made by every one of our cells and can either feed pathways that create disease or restore health. Fish oils are also important for supporting the cardiovascular system and for developing the brain and nervous system.

DOSAGE: *Take up to 2 Tbsp of flax oil daily and/or up to 3000 mg fish oil daily with a minimum of 800 mg EPA and 400 mg DHA.*

## L-Arginine
L-arginine has been reported to increase sperm motility, quality and count. It also helps with improving blood flow to the uterus increasing fertility.

DOSAGE: *800–1600 mg daily*

## CoQ10 – Ubiquinone

CoQ10 is a potent antioxidant that helps improve sperm motility. A recent animal study showed positive effects, after CoQ10 supplementation, on rejuvenating egg quality. This may prove to be a promising treatment in infertility cases.

DOSAGE: *100 mg daily*

## Lycopene

Lycopene is found in high concentrations in the testes where it may help prevent free radical damage to the sperm. Low levels of lycopene have also been found in infertile men.

DOSAGE: *4 mg daily*

## Maca – *Lepidium meyeii*

Maca is a root vegetable cultivated in the Peruvian Andes that belongs to the brassica family. Maca is rich in amino acids, iodine, iron, and magnesium. Traditionally, Maca root has been used for its fertility- and libido-enhancing properties. Studies have shown improvements in seminal volume, sperm count, and sperm motility. Maca also increases energy and may be useful for supporting the body's stress response and healthy adrenal function.

DOSAGE: *2–4 capsules daily of* **Ultimate Maca Energy**™, *1 tsp daily of* **Maca-Punch Platinum Liquid Extract**™ *or 1 Tbsp of* **Ultimate Maca Energy**™ *Powder*

## Probiotics – *Lactobacillus acidophilus* and *Bifidobacterium* spp.

Probiotics are known to have an important role in the maintenance of normal flora in the gastrointestinal and urinary tract. Probiotics also support optimal immune function as 70% of our immune cells do reside in our gut!

DOSAGE: *at least 10 billion CFU daily with food*

## Chaste Tree Berry - *Vitex agnus castus*

Chaste Tree Berry (*Vitex*) has an effect on the hypothalamus/hypophysis axis. It increases luteinizing hormone from the pituitary gland that subsequently favours progesterone. This herb helps modulate prolactin levels which may improve fertility.

DOSAGE: *175–250 mg daily*

## Dong Quai – *Angelica sinensis*

Dong Quai is a Chinese herb that can improve uterine tonicity as well as help regulate hormones and improve irregular menstruation.

DOSAGE: *200 mg daily*

## Rhodiola – *Rhodiola rosea*

The herb Rhodiola is an important adaptogen that is useful during times of stress to support healthy adrenal function and stress response. It also may enhance fertility. A study of 40 women with a loss of menstrual cycle were given 100 mg twice daily for two weeks. Normal menses was restored in 25 women, 11 of whom became pregnant. Hopefully more research will be conducted on this herb for fertility in the near future.

DOSAGE: *200 mg daily*

## Thyroid Support – *ThyroSense*®

Hypothyroidism can be a key cause for infertility in men and women. Couples who are having difficulty conceiving should have a full thyroid panel done to rule out low thyroid function.

DOSAGE: *2 capsules twice daily*

## Adrenal Support – *AdrenaSense®*

Stress is a known factor in couples that are having difficulty conceiving. The adrenal glands are the body's main stress responders and poor adrenal function can be associated with hormone imbalance and thus poor fertility. Support those adrenal glands!

DOSAGE: *1 capsule one to three times daily*

## Liver Support – *EstroSense®*

EstroSense® is a unique formula that combines indole-3-carbinol, sulforaphane, DIM, calcium-d-glucarate, milk thistle and potent antioxidants (curcumin, rosemary extract, lycopene, green tea extract) to help maintain healthy hormone levels by targeting estrogen metabolism. It may be helpful for women who are experiencing irregular menstruation, no menstruation, PMS or heavy periods.

DOSAGE: *3 capsules twice daily*

## Other Beneficial Herbs

Herbs to consider:

- Blue Cohosh – *Caulophyllum thalictroides*
- Crampbark – *Viburnum opulus*
- False Unicorn – *Chamaelerium luteum*
- Squaw Vine – *Mitchella repens*
- Red Clover – *Trifolium pretense*
- Tribulus - *Tribulus terrestris*
- Red Raspberry – *Rubus idaeus.*

## CONVENTIONAL MEDICINE

### Fertility Drugs

Fertility drugs are the main treatment for women who are infertile due to ovulation disorders. These medications regulate or induce ovulation.

Commonly used fertility drugs include:

- **Clomiphene citrate (Clomid).** This drug stimulates ovulation in women who have polycystic ovary syndrome (PCOS) or other ovulatory disorders. It causes the pituitary gland to release more FSH and LH, which stimulate the growth of an ovarian follicle containing an egg. It can be taken after sexual intercourse or injection of sperm.
- **Metformin (Glucophage).** This drug is commonly used in women with PCOS and insulin resistance, which can be suspected causes of infertility.
- **Bromocriptine (Parlodel).** This medication is for women whose ovulation cycles are irregular due to elevated levels of prolactin, the hormone that stimulates milk production in new mothers. Elevated prolactin levels are often seen in women with PCOS. Bromocriptine inhibits prolactin production.

## Surgery

Surgery may be indicated for those women who have scar tissue on the ovaries, fallopian tubes or uterus, or have blockages in the fallopian tubes.

## *In vitro* fertilization (IVF)

IVF involves the retrieval of mature eggs from a woman and subsequently fertilizing them with male sperm in a laboratory culture dish. Two to three days later, multiple eggs are implanted in the woman's uterus. This procedure may be repeated several times over a period of months until a successful pregnancy occurs.

# CHAPTER 13

# INTERSTITIAL CYSTITIS

Interstitial cystitis (also known as painful bladder, leaky bladder or irritative bladder syndrome) is a chronic, multifactorial syndrome characterized by a combination of pelvic pain, pressure, or discomfort in the bladder and pelvic region, often associated with urinary frequency and urgency.

It is estimated that 450,000 people in the US and 50,000 in Canada have interstitial cystitis (IC) with 90% being women. IC is frequently misdiagnosed as a urinary tract infection and patients may go years without a correct diagnosis. This condition often occurs around age 30 or 40, although it has been reported in younger people.

## RISK FACTORS

The following risk factors may be associated with a higher risk of IC and include:

- **Sex** – women are diagnosed with IC far more often than men. Men can have identical symptoms to IC but these are more commonly associated with inflammation of the prostate gland (prostatitis).
- **Age** – most people with IC are diagnosed in their 30s and 40s.
- **Chronic Disorders** – IC may be associated with other chronic pain syndromes such as irritable bowel syndrome, rheumatoid arthritis,

hay fever, asthma, hysterectomy, fibromyalgia or allergies to foods and medications.

## SIGNS and SYMPTOMS

Signs and symptoms of IC vary from person to person and may be triggered by menstruation, prolonged sitting, stress, exercise or sexual activity. Some common signs and symptoms include:

- Pain in the pelvis or between the vagina and anus in women or between the scrotum and anus in men
- Chronic pelvic pain
- A persistent, urgent need to urinate
- Frequent urination, often in small amounts, throughout the day and night
- Pain during sexual intercourse.

Although signs and symptoms of IC resemble those of a chronic urinary tract infection, urine cultures are usually free of bacteria.

## CAUSES

Several theories have been proposed for IC involving structural, hormonal, neurological, autoimmune, lymphatic, infectious and psychological factors.

### Bladder Epithelial Permeability

The bladder epithelium contains sulphated glycosaminoglycans (GAGs) that, when healthy, protect the bladder from toxins, microorganisms and carcinogens which may damage the bladder wall. It is suggested that individuals diagnosed with IC have a breakdown of this protective layer leading to changes in permeability, stimulation of pain receptors and inflammation. This permeable layer allows toxic components from the urine to penetrate and irritate and bladder.

## Neurological

"Substance P" is an inflammatory mediator released by nerves in the peripheral nervous system. Increased levels of substance P have been found in the urine of women with IC, with concentrations dependent on the severity of pain.

Injury to peripheral nerves from prior urinary tract infections (UTIs), hysterectomy or childbirth may also lead to an increase in pain impulses from the bladder causing inflammation and bladder ulceration.

## Mast Cell Activation

Mast cells play a key role in the inflammatory process. When activated, they release histamine, prostaglandins and other substances that may affect the bladder. The theory is that mast cells are activated in response to the "leaky" bladder wall and this creates more inflammation.

## The Role of Estrogens

It has been reported that 40% of IC patients, experience an exacerbation of symptoms, particularly around the time of ovulation. This has led to the proposal that estrogen plays a role in determining the intensity of inflammation within the bladder by activating mast cells.

## Autoimmune

Some researchers suggest that IC is similar to an autoimmune disease or process due to the presence of specific bladder autoantibodies.

## Inflammation

Inflammation is a strong theory as a cause of IC since a significant level of inflammatory mediators, such as Interleukin-6, are found in the bladder.

## Infection

The symptoms of IC are very similar to bacterial cystitis but urine samples often demonstrate no evidence of an infection. The possibility that there is an infectious cause is up for debate but the thought is that very small amounts of microorganisms may be able to persist in the bladder wall.

## TESTS and DIAGNOSIS

An initial evaluation of IC includes a patient history, physical exam and review of symptoms. Key diagnostic symptoms are: bladder and pelvic pain or discomfort, urinary urgency or frequency, symptoms that persist for more than six weeks and negative results of lab tests checking for urinary tract or other infections.

IC patients often have overlapping symptoms related to other pelvic diseases and therefore it is important to rule out conditions such as: urinary tract and genital tract infections, tumors of the urinary or gastrointestinal tract, and endometriosis. Many patients with IC are treated over and over with courses of antibiotics for urinary tract infections before being definitely diagnosed.

A pelvic exam and urinalysis are often performed first, followed by a cystoscopy in which the doctor looks for inflammation or any ulceration in the bladder wall. Sometimes a test called the potassium sensitivity test, also known as Parson's Test, will be used. It involves inserting two solutions – water and potassium chloride – into the bladder, one at a time. On a scale of 0 to 5, the patient's pain and urgency is recorded and typically those who have IC will report more pain when the potassium is instilled.

## PREVENTION and TREATMENT – Dietary and Lifestyle

## FOOD FACTORS

Many individuals battling IC find avoiding certain foods and beverages helpful in preventing flare-ups. *The Interstitial Cystitis Association* suggests that the following foods should be avoided:

- Aged cheeses
- Alcohol
- Artificial sweeteners – aspartame, sucralose

- Carbonated drinks
- Chilies/spicy foods
- Chocolate
- Citrus juices
- Coffee
- Cranberry juice
- Fava and lima beans
- Meats that are cured, processed, smoked, canned, aged or that contain nitrites
- Fruits: plums, apple, banana, prune, cantaloupe, peach, strawberry, pineapple, grapes
- Nuts except: almonds, cashews, and pine nuts
- Onions
- Rye bread
- MSG
- Sour cream
- Sourdough bread
- Soy
- Tea
- Tofu
- Tomatoes
- Yogurt.

Not all individuals with IC are sensitive to the same foods. It may be helpful to test for allergies using an ELISA testing method through a Naturopathic Doctor or complementary health care practitioner. An elimination/challenge diet can also be tried to determine food sensitivities.

## LIFESTYLE TIPS
- Avoid all processed, refined foods and those with artificial sweeteners, colours etc.
- Try to wear loose clothing to minimize pressure on the abdomen and pelvic region.

- Reduce stress! Practice meditation, yoga, deep breathing or treat yourself to a massage once a month.
- Try pelvic floor exercises. Gently stretching and strengthening the pelvic floor muscles, possibly with the help from a physical therapist, may reduce muscle spasms.
- Don't smoke!
- Exercise at least 30 to 40 minutes a minimum of three times per week. The ideal routine is a combination of aerobic and stretching/ weight training.

## KEY SUPPLEMENTS

### L-Arginine

L-arginine is a precursor to nitric oxide, which plays a role in the relaxation of the urinary tract smooth muscle. There have been conflicting studies with L-arginine and it may not work for everyone. It is probably best to try L-arginine on its own before combining it with other treatment options.

DOSAGE: *500 mg three times daily*

### Quercetin

A high concentration of activated mast cells has been found in the bladder of those individuals with interstitial cystitis. The flavonoid, quercetin has anti-inflammatory properties and helps inhibit mast cell activity as well.

DOSAGE: *500–1000 mg twice daily*

### N-Acetyl Glucosamine

The bladder wall is lined by a layer of glycosaminoglycans (GAGs), which act as a barrier between the tissues of the bladder wall and urine. Individuals with IC often have an abnormal bladder wall which is permeable. Therefore, supplementing with N-acetyl glucosamine may be helpful in repairing the bladder epithelium.

DOSAGE: *500 mg twice daily*

## Vitamin C – Buffered

Vitamin C is an immune booster that could assist in the treatment of IC by reducing inflammation, killing any microorganisms and modulating the immune system so that it is in healthy balance.

DOSAGE: *1000-2000 mg daily or to bowel tolerance*

## Plant Sterols – *ImmunoCare™*

Plant sterols are immune modulators, meaning that in cases where the immune system is "overactive", as in autoimmune diseases, they will help lower that immune response and bring it back into balance. Plant sterols also help decrease inflammatory cytokines that may be associated with IC. As well, they support the stress response by maintaining healthy cortisol levels.

DOSAGE: *1 capsule daily*

## Corn Silk – *Zea mays*

Corn silk possesses anti-inflammatory properties and has been used for numerous urinary conditions.

DOSAGE: *300 mg three times daily or drink in tea form*

## Probiotics - *Lactobacillus acidophilus* and *Bifidobacterium* spp.

Probiotics are known to play an important role in the maintenance of normal flora in the gastrointestinal and urinary tract. Probiotics also support optimal immune function as 70% of our immune cells do reside in our gut!

DOSAGE: *at least 10 billion CFU daily with food*

## Flaxseed Oil and/or Pure Fish Oil

Essential fatty acids in the form of flaxseed or uncontaminated fish oil decrease the formation of PGE2, a type of prostaglandin that acts as a messenger molecule to promote inflammatory pathways in the body. Prostaglandins are made by every one of our cells and can either feed pathways that create disease or restore health.

DOSAGE: *Take up to 2 tbsp of flax oil daily and/or up to 3000 mg fish oil daily with a minimum of 1000 mg EPA and 600 mg DHA.*

## Liver Support – *EstroSense®*

EstroSense® is a unique formula that combines indole-3-carbinol, DIM, calcium-d-glucarate, sulforaphane, milk thistle and potent anti-oxidants (curcumin, rosemary extract, lycopene, green tea extract) to help maintain healthy hormone levels by targeting estrogen metabolism. As estrogen may be a trigger for individuals with IC, supporting healthy estrogen levels might help in reducing potential flare-ups.

DOSAGE: *3 capsules twice daily*

## CONVENTIONAL MEDICINE

### Oral Medications

Oral medications may improve the signs and symptoms of interstitial cystitis. These include:

- Ibuprofen (Advil, Motrin), naproxen (Aleve) and other nonsteroidal anti-inflammatory drugs, to relieve pain
- Tricyclic antidepressants, such as amitriptyline or imipramine (Tofranil), to help relax the bladder and block pain
- Antihistamines, such as diphenhydramine (Benadryl) and loratadine (Claritin), which may reduce urinary urgency and frequency and relieve other symptoms
- Pentosan (Elmiron) is the only oral drug approved by the Food and

Drug Administration specifically for interstitial cystitis. How it works is unknown, but it may restore the inner surface of the bladder, which protects the bladder wall from substances in urine that could irritate it. It may take two to four months before you begin to feel pain relief and up to six months to experience a decrease in urinary frequency. Side effects include minor gastrointestinal disturbances and possible hair loss, which reverses when you stop taking the drug. It only shows an efficacy rate of about a 30%.

## Medications Inserted into the Bladder

The prescription medication dimethyl sulfoxide or DMSO is placed into the bladder through a catheter weekly or biweekly to help reduce inflammation and prevent muscle contractions that cause frequency, urgency and pain.

## Nerve Stimulation

Transcutaneous electrical nerve stimulation (TENS) uses mild electrical pulses to relieve pelvic pain and in some cases, to reduce urinary frequency.

## Bladder Distension

Bladder distension involves stretching the bladder with water or gas and may provide temporary improvement in symptoms for individuals with IC.

## Surgery

Surgery is often considered a last resort and most surgical procedures are associated with a high rate of relapse, pain and additional surgeries.

CHAPTER 14

# MENOPAUSE

Menopause represents a major transitional period in a woman's life. Most women enter menopause between the ages of 45 and 50. The term "menopause" is derived from *meno* (month, menses) plus *pausis* (pause, cessation) which is the true definition of menopause - one year with no menstrual cycle. Peri-menopause is the period immediately before menopause, which typically starts with changes in the menstrual cycle and ends 12 months after the final menstrual period. On average, 70-80 percent of women will experience mild to moderate symptoms, while 10-15 percent will suffer severe symptoms. These typically last between two and eight years, although some women may report experiencing symptoms for longer.

Common symptoms include:

- Hot flashes
- Night sweats
- Sleep disturbances
- Anxiety and depression
- Vaginal dryness
- Irregular periods
- Joint pain
- Brain fog and memory problems

- Fatigue
- Sore breasts
- Headaches
- Decreased libido
- Bladder incontinence
- Heart palpitations
- Weight gain
- Recurrent bladder or vaginal infections
- Increased risk of heart disease (see **Heart Disease and Stroke** Chapter)
- Increased risk of osteoporosis (see **Osteoporosis** Chapter).

During this time, women experience a decreased production of sex hormones by the ovaries and the adrenal glands. Fat cells take over and become the primary sources for sex hormone production (see **Adrenal Fatigue** Chapter). Remember that the adrenal glands are the two small glands that sit on top of each kidney and support the body's ability to cope with, or adapt to, stress. Therefore, the stress of everyday life as well as the transition into menopause no doubt creates much strain on the adrenal glands. Many women have "stressed" or "fatigued" adrenal glands long before they reach menopause, making their menopausal symptoms much harder to cope with.

## HOT FLASHES
Hot flashes are sudden feelings of warmth that are usually most intense over the face, neck and chest but can also progress toward the feet with an entire body sensation experienced by some women. They can last a few seconds to a few minutes with concurrent symptoms such as palpitations, anxiety, irritability and night sweats. Some women may experience hot flashes every hour. Hot flashes can begin prior to the last menstrual period with nearly 60% of women reporting them before any menstrual changes are experienced. Patterns may change, with some women experiencing hot flashes less frequently and intensely over time while others continue to experience discomfort well into their later

years. One of the major complaints associated with hot flashes is insomnia, which can have a domino effect on the woman's overall quality of life. In cooler environments, hot flashes are fewer, less intense, and shorter in duration.

## Risk Factors and Triggers for Hot Flashes

There are many proposed theories as to why some women report more severe symptoms of hot flashing than others. The common origin, however, seems to stem from an imbalance in the central thermoregulatory centre likely due to decreased levels of estrogen. A drop in estrogen can trigger changes in levels or function of the neurotransmitter norepinephrine, which results in dilation of blood vessels, flushing and sweating. Specific prostaglandins (chemical messengers), known as PGE2 and PGF2a, stimulate the hypothalamus (part of the brain that controls temperature) whereby inflammation and blood circulation is increased, promoting flushing. Hot flashes usually coincide with surges of LH (a hormone produced by the pituitary gland). Other neurotransmitters such as endorphins, serotonin and GABA will modulate the release of LH. A disruption in their action (stress) on the hypothalamus may cause LH to rise thus producing a hot flash.

Other possible triggers or risk factors include:

- Physical inactivity
- Adrenal exhaustion
- Stress/overwork
- Hot drinks
- Spicy foods
- Alcohol
- Foods containing histamine such as cheese or wine
- Chocolate
- Caffeine
- Smoking
- Red meat, dairy fat, peanuts, shellfish
- Hot weather

- Menopause before the age of 52
- Onset of menstrual period before age 12
- History of irregular periods
- High levels of TSH during menopause (low thyroid)
- Tamoxifen, aromatase inhibitors used in breast cancer patients.

 **FACT – Did You Know?**

Acupuncture can be very effective in reducing menopausal symptoms such as hot flashes and night sweats. One study found that 6 to 14 acupuncture treatments twice weekly, reduced hot flashes by over 50%!

## VAGINAL DRYNESS and THINNING

Vaginal dryness is a common problem for women during and after menopause. Estrogen is responsible for the thickened, elastic and lubricated tissue of the vagina. When estrogen levels decline during menopause, the cells of the vagina lose collagen, fat and the ability to retain water. As a result, they lose tone, become flattened, thin and dry. The thinner tissue and dryness can cause more irritation making intercourse uncomfortable or painful. The "good" bacteria that normally reside in the vagina also decrease in number during menopause, increasing the risk of vaginal or bladder infections.

## INSOMNIA

Approximately 61% of postmenopausal women have sleep problems which can then lead to impaired cognitive function, fatigue, depression and reduced quality of life. In addition, hot flushes and night sweats, which affect 75 to 85% of postmenopausal women, can also affect sleep quality. Some women will have difficulty falling asleep and others may find themselves waking up multiple times in the night and not being able to go back to sleep.

## MOOD SWINGS, DEPRESSION AND ANXIETY

Sleepless nights may exaggerate moods, depression and anxiety in some menopausal women. During menopause, there is a fluctuation of hormones adding much stress to the body. With the body trying to cope with this transition and the adrenal glands trying to support the on-going hormonal changes, moods can shift significantly leading to depression, anxiety, panic and irritability. When they reach menopause, most women already have their "tanks half full" from day-to-day stressors and life in general. This can greatly influence how the body copes with the stress of going through menopause. The thyroid gland (see **Hypothyroidism** Chapter) also greatly influences moods, depression and anxiety and should be checked along with adrenal gland function (see **Adrenal Fatigue** Chapter) to support a smooth transition through menopause.

### *PREVENTION and TREATMENT – Dietary and Lifestyle*

### FOOD FACTORS

Nutrition and diet can greatly influence menopause and menopausal symptoms. One of the most important dietary recommendations for all menopausal women may be to increase foods that are high in phyto-estrogens. Phytoestrogens are plant versions of the human hormone estrogen. They're considered to be weak estrogenic compounds with an average of about two% of the strength of estrogens. They can be beneficial when estrogen levels are either too high or too low. When metabolized, they bind on the same cellular sites as do estrogens, altering estrogenic effects. The three main classes of phytoestrogens are isoflavones, lignans and coumestans. Isoflavones are the most widely studied class of phytoestrogens, with genistein and daidzein providing most of the data. The best food sources of phytoestrogens are non-genetically engineered organic soybeans, flax seeds, oats, rye, lentils, fennel, chickpeas, alfalfa and sesame. Much research shows that women in Asia experience less menopausal symptoms because their diet contains a higher concentration of phytoestrogens, compared to women who adopt a North American diet.

There has been much controversy recently about soy and concerns about its safety. These concerns are based on its weak estrogenic and hormonal effects. Several studies have concluded that Asian women who consume a traditional low-fat, high-soy diet have a four- to six-fold lower risk of developing breast cancer. The dietary phytoestrogens have also been shown to inhibit cancer growth by competing with estradiol for the type II estrogen binding sites. The type and frequency of soy consumed is also important. My recommendation to patients is to choose organic, non-GMO forms of soy as well as fermented soy products such as tempeh or miso. I recommend eating soy in moderation, meaning between 50 to 150 mg of isoflavones (phytoestrogens) daily. For example, one cup of regular soymilk contains 30 mg and half a cup of tofu will contain 35 mg of isoflavones. Before making any conclusions about soy, it's important to remember that every woman is different and what may work for one woman may not for the other. Women with soy allergies may have difficulty digesting it.

Our North American diet is typically deficient in essential fatty acids (EFAs) which are very important in many health conditions, ranging from inflammation and PMS to menopausal symptoms. Supplementing with essential fatty acids from flax or better yet, from a good quality fish oil rich in omega-3s, will help with various menopausal symptoms. A woman's risk of heart disease and stroke significantly increases after menopause. Even more reason to include those healthy fats!

To reduce stress on the liver, enjoy foods fresh from the tree or plucked from the earth rather than packaged in a box or can. Spicy foods, sugar, hot foods and beverages as well as caffeine can trigger hot flashes, so keep intake of these items to a minimum. Dairy products and red meats have also been associated with an increase in hot flashes.

A diet rich in cruciferous vegetables (broccoli, Brussels sprouts, cauliflower, cabbage and kale) contain indole-3-carbinol and sulforaphane, important nutrients for maintaining balanced hormones in the liver while reducing the risk of breast cancer.

Boosting the amount of fibre in the diet is critical to prevent constipation and promote the transport of harmful, excess estrogens from the body. Adequate fibre and healthy proteins help stabilize blood sugar and alleviate some hormone fluctuations. New research shows that not only does a low Glycemic Index (GI) diet help to improve blood glucose levels, but it also helps people reduce food intake (possibly by making us feel full longer) and contributes to weight loss. Include low GI foods as part of a regular dietary plan (see **Appendix**).

Limit salt intake, which can increase the amount of calcium secreted in urine. This is a key concern considering the increased risk of bone thinning at menopause. Instead, season food with herbs, spices, garlic and onions.

## LIFESTYLE TIPS

- To reduce hot flashes and night sweats, keep your bedroom cool. Dress in layers so you can always be a comfortable temperature.
- Wear only cotton and natural fabrics on your body; use only cotton bed sheets.
- Avoid very hot liquids and foods, and instead opt for cool water when a hot flash begins. Avoid alcohol.
- To reduce insomnia, train your body to anticipate sleep. Create a bedtime routine – have a warm bath, read a book, enjoy some tea containing chamomile flowers, passionflower herb, skullcap herb, valerian and hibiscus flowers. Avoid stimulating activities such as watching TV or surfing the internet.
- Practice Kegel exercises to improve muscle tone and blood circulation to the vagina and bladder.
- Make time for stress-releasing activities like massage, yoga, hiking, painting, and journaling – whatever helps you relax and unwind. Support your adrenal glands (see **Adrenal Fatigue** Chapter).
- Eliminate food sensitivities, as hot flashes can be reduced by 50% if sensitive foods are removed.
- Eliminate carbonated beverages as too much phosphorus competes with calcium absorption. Carbonation causes the body's pH to become acidic thus increasing bone resorption leading to osteoporosis.
- Try to consume organic meats wherever possible (no hormones, by-products or antibiotics). The estrogen in animal meats will bind tightly to estrogen receptors encouraging breast cancer.

- Eliminate caffeine, cigarettes, alcohol and sugar. These can create an acidic environment in the body and thus leach calcium out of the bone to balance the body's pH.
- Minimize exposure to exogenous estrogens: HRT, pesticides, herbicides, plastics, and hormones used to fatten livestock and promote milk production (meats and dairy).
- EXERCISE! Aerobic and weight-bearing to improve heart function, decrease bone loss, give relief from hot flashes, reduce BP, decrease cholesterol, increase mood and energy.

## KEY SUPPLEMENTS

### Black Cohosh – *Cimicifuga racemosa*

Black cohosh has been used for a variety of women's health conditions, especially for the treatment of menopausal symptoms such as hot flashes and night sweats. Clinical and observational practice suggests black cohosh may be approximately 25 to 30% more effective than placebo for menopausal symptoms, including hot flashes. In one of the largest studies, 629 women with menopausal complaints received a liquid standardized extract of black cohosh of 40 drops twice per day for six to eight weeks. As early as four weeks after beginning the therapy, improvements in menopausal symptoms was seen in 80% of the women. After six to eight weeks, menopausal symptoms completely disappeared in 50 percent of the women. Studies have concluded black cohosh is non-toxic, non-mutagenic, non-carcinogenic and suitable for long-term treatment. Its use in Europe for more than 40 years in over 1.5 million cases demonstrates excellent tolerability and low risk of side effects. The German Commission E has approved the use of black cohosh for menopausal symptoms at daily doses of 40-200 mg. The current rec-

> **Body/Mind Connection**
> Menopausal symptoms are associated with a fear of being unwanted or a fear of aging. Focus instead on being peaceful with changing cycles and loving yourself.

ommended dose is 40-80 mg per day. At least four to twelve weeks of treatment may be required before therapeutic benefits are apparent.

DOSAGE: *40-200 mg daily*

## Chaste Tree Berry - *Vitex agnus castus*

The effect of Chaste tree berry is on the hypothalamus/hypophysis axis. It increases luteinizing hormone and has an effect favouring progesterone. Many women when transitioning into menopause will experience irregular periods, either too heavy or too frequent. Chaste tree berry is a beneficial herb to help normalize and regulate periods during perimenopause. Women will also experience a sudden drop in progesterone when transitioning into menopause, which can cause mood swings, breast swelling, low libido and the above symptoms of irregular periods. Chaste tree berry may ease and prevent these symptoms during the hormonal shifts of menopause.

DOSAGE: *80-160 mg daily*

## Dong Quai

Dong Quai is known as the "female ginseng" and traditionally, has been indicated for menstrual disorders and as a supportive herb for menopausal complaints. Its effectiveness in relieving hot flashes may be due to a combination of its ability to stabilize blood vessels and its antispasmodic effects. It also contains ferulic acid which as has been shown to decrease hot flashes.

DOSAGE: *100-200 mg daily*

## Hesperidin

The flavonoid hesperidin, from citrus fruit, is known to improve vascular integrity and decrease capillary permeability thereby strengthening blood vessels walls, reducing hot flashes and improving leg cramps.

DOSAGE: *150–300 mg daily*

## Gamma-Oryzanol

Gamma-oryzanol is isolated from rice bran oil and contains a compound called ferulic acid that is responsible for its antioxidant properties. Ferulic acid may protect against various inflammatory conditions and has been shown to be effective in reducing menopausal hot flashes.

DOSAGE: *150–300 mg daily*
***All the above nutrients are found in **MenoSense®**, an excellent formula for the relief of menopausal symptoms such as hot flashes, night sweats, and insomnia.

DOSAGE: *2 capsules twice daily*
*Note: Can be used in conjunction with hormone replacement therapy (synthetic or bio-identical) or to help wean off of HRT.*

## Vitamin C

Vitamin C is a potent antioxidant that supports blood vessels, collagen formation, immunity, heart health and other health conditions. It may also help to decrease harmful PGE2 prostaglandins that increase inflammation and hot flashes in menopausal women.

DOSAGE: *1000–2000 mg daily or to bowel tolerance*

## Vitamin E – Mixed Tocopherols

Research on vitamin E for the reduction of hot flashes, mood swings, palpitations, dizziness, anxiety and vaginal dryness suggests that supplementation may be beneficial. Studies as early as the 1940s found doses of 50-400 IU effective in decreasing hot flashes and other menopausal complaints over placebo. One study showed an increase in blood supply to the vaginal wall when taken for at least four weeks.

DOSAGE: *400–800 IU daily orally or insert vaginally or apply topically to relieve vaginal dryness and improve lubrication.*

## Vitamin B Complex
The B vitamins are important for liver detoxification and the metabolism of excess and harmful estrogens as well as help support the stress response and adrenal glands.

DOSAGE: *50–100 mg daily*

## Vitamin B6
Vitamin B6 is involved in serotonin production as well as other important brain neurotransmitters and therefore, may be helpful in lifting moods and helping depression. Women who are taking conjugated equine estrogen (Premarin) or the birth control pill are often deficient in vitamin B6 and should be supplemented. A Vitamin B6 deficiency can often cause irritability and insomnia. Thus supplementation may prove helpful for various menopausal symptoms.

DOSAGE: *50–200 mg daily*

## Calcium/Magnesium with Vitamin D
Calcium and magnesium both help improve relaxation and sleep. They maintain healthy bone density along with other bone builders including vitamin K, boron, silicon and manganese among others (see **Osteoporosis** Chapter).

DOSAGE: *1000–1500 mg of calcium citrate/malate, 500–750 mg of magnesium citrate/bisglycinate and 2000–4000 IU of vitamin D.*

## Probiotics - *Lactobacillus acidophilus* and *Bifidobacterium* spp.
Probiotics are known to play an important role in the maintenance of normal flora in the gastrointestinal tract. They also help with the detoxification and binding of harmful estrogens in the digestive tract and eliminate them from the body through the colon.

DOSAGE: *at least 10 billion CFU daily with food.*

## Pure Fish Oil/Flaxseed Oil (Omega-3 Fatty Acids)

Essential fatty acids, in the form of uncontaminated pure fish oil, block the formation of PGE2 which is a messenger molecule that helps increase inflammatory pathways in the body. They are very helpful in reducing pain and inflammation, hot flashes and preventing heart disease.

DOSAGE: *Take up to two Tbsp of flax oil daily and/or 3000 mg fish oil daily with a minimum of 800 mg EPA and 400 mg DHA.*

## St. John's Wort

St. John's Wort is one of the most widely researched herbs for the treatment of depression. Its mechanism of action seems to improve the activity of both serotonin and GABA, which help lift mood and relax the brain and nervous system. Menopausal women often have major hormonal fluctuations that can deeply affect brain chemistry thus causing depression, irritability, anger or anxiety.

DOSAGE: *300 mg one to three times daily*
*\*Note: St. John's Wort may cause photosensitivity in some individuals and therefore, be careful out in the sun. Also, it should not be taken with pharmaceutical anti-depressants such as SSRIs or during chemotherapy.*

## Melatonin – *SleepSense*®

Melatonin helps to maintain the body's circadian rhythm, an internal 24-hour "clock" that plays a critical role in regulating when we fall asleep and when we wake up. The body produces more melatonin when it is dark and its production decreases when it is light. Being exposed to bright lights too late in the evening can disrupt the melatonin production.

There is also a relationship with cortisol and stress. During chronic stress, cortisol levels are high in the evening – exactly when they are supposed to be at their lowest. This lowers melatonin levels thus disrupting sleep. Hormonal changes during menopause often add more stress on the adrenal glands and affect other hormones such as melatonin, which is another excellent reason why adrenal support is so important during menopause.

DOSAGE: *3 mg tablets one to three tablets dissolved under the tongue at least 30 minutes before bed.*

## 5-HTP – *HappySense*®

5-HTP is another supplement that may benefit sleep as well as moods such as anxiety and depression. 5-HTP is the precursor to serotonin, which is then converted into melatonin.

DOSAGE: *50 or 100 mg 1–2 caplets one to three times daily. MAXIMUM 600 mg daily.*

## GABA – Gamma-Aminobutyric Acid

GABA is a neurotransmitter that works like a "brake" during times of runaway stress. Stress excites the nervous system, causing irritability, restlessness, anxiety, insomnia and movement disorders. GABA helps to regulate brain excitability.

DOSAGE: *100–500 mg daily*

## Maca

Maca has been used in Peru for thousands of years. It has proven to be useful for boosting energy levels, supporting the production of estrogen and testosterone, improving libido and providing relief of some menopausal symptoms. Maca seems to act on the hypothalamus and pituitary, two key players in hormone balance.

DOSAGE: *2–4 capsules daily of* **Ultimate Maca Energy**™*, 1 tsp daily of* **MacaPunch Platinum Liquid Extract**™ *or 1 tbsp of* **Ultimate Maca Energy Powder**™

## Adrenal Support – *AdrenaSense®*

Supporting the adrenal glands before and during menopause seems to be the missing link for most women. The adrenal glands are key players in menopause and take over the production of sex hormones when the ovaries shut down. Healthy adrenal gland function is therefore critically important to help women transition into menopause naturally and easier.

DOSAGE: *1–3 capsules daily*

## Thyroid Support – *ThyroSense®*

During menopause, the thyroid gland and hormones often become unstable so thyroid gland support may be indicated. Some common low thyroid symptoms include difficulty losing weight, cold intolerance, fatigue and brittle hair and nails.

DOSAGE: *Take 2 capsules twice daily.*

## Liver Support – *EstroSense®*

Increasing liver detoxification is vitally important to the elimination of harmful estrogens and maintaining healthy hormone balance.

Important supplements such as milk thistle, turmeric, indole-3-carbinol, sulforaphane, calcium-d-glucarate, DIM, green tea extract, lycopene and rosemary extract help support estrogen metabolism through the liver and bind harmful by-products thus promoting their elimination from the body.

DOSAGE: *3 capsules two times daily*

## BIO-IDENTICAL HORMONE THERAPY

Bio-identical hormone therapy uses synthesized hormones that are exact chemical replicas of those produced in the human body. The bio-identical hormones include: estrone, estradiol, estriol, progesterone, testosterone, and dehydroespiandrosterone (DHEA).

Available bio-identical hormones that may be prescribed for hot flashes and other menopausal symptoms include bi-est (80% estriol and 20% estradiol), tri-est (80% estriol, 10% estradiol and 10% estrone) and progesterone.

## Natural Progesterone Cream

Natural progesterone cream can be used alone for the treatment of hot flashes if estrogen is not tolerated.

*Dosing for Perimenopausal Women*

Days 1 to 7: do not use progesterone cream during menstrual period
Days 8 to 21: ¼ tsp twice daily
Days 22 to 28: ¼-1/2 tsp twice daily

*Dosing for Menopausal or Postmenopausal Women*

On a continuous basis, take ¼ tsp daily.

*Note: Progesterone cream should be applied to the inner arms, inner thighs or labia of the vagina. Location should be rotated to avoid saturated progesterone receptors in the body.

## Estriol Cream for Vaginal Dryness

Estriol is considered safe and the weakest of all three estrogens. It is a protective estrogen against breast cancer and other potential estrogen dominant conditions. It can be useful for vaginal dryness, improves sexual intercourse and prevents bladder and vaginal infections. It can be used as a topical cream or suppository.

I use bio-identical hormones in my practice as a last resort, once the above therapies have been exhausted. I also determine its use, form and dose depending on each individual woman's case and the severity of her symptoms. To determine estrogen dosages (Bi-Est/Tri-Est), please seek the guidance from an ND or a complementary MD.

## CONVENTIONAL MEDICINE

Hormone replacement therapy (HRT) has been a popular course of treatment for most women with menopausal symptoms, but the decision to use HRT is a difficult one. Many studies have investigated some of the dangerous side effects of HRT including the increased risk in breast cancer, cardiovascular disease, stroke and blood clots. It is important to discuss the pros and cons with your health care provider to determine the best treatment plan for your individual menopausal symptoms. Some of the most common conventional approaches are discussed below.

### Hormone Therapy

Estrogen and progesterone are the hormones often prescribed by medical doctors to reduce hot flashes. These synthetic hormones are not identical to a woman's own estrogen and progesterone and therefore, can create damaging and harmful by-products once metabolized through the liver. Conjugated equine estrogens (Premarin) are derived from the urine of pregnant mares.

Many women are choosing bio-identical hormones or other natural treatment options. As mentioned above, synthetic hormone therapy has been associated with some dangerous side effects such as increased risk of breast cancer, cardiovascular disease, stroke and blood clots. Other adverse effects of HRT may include headaches, nausea, water retention, phlebitis, breast tenderness and irritability.

As an alternative for women who can't take estrogen, some doctors prescribe progesterone alone to help control hot flashes.

### Antidepressants

Low doses of certain antidepressants may decrease hot flashes. Antidepressants may also be prescribed to help with stabilizing moods such as anxiety and depression.

Examples include:

- Venlafaxine (Effexor)
- Paroxetine (Paxil)
- Fluoxetine (Prozac).

However, these medications aren't as effective as hormone therapy for severe hot flashes and may cause side effects, such as nausea, dizziness, weight gain or sexual dysfunction.

## Gabapentin

Gabapentin is an anti-seizure medication that's moderately effective in reducing hot flashes, particularly for women who have symptoms at night. Side effects can include drowsiness, dizziness and headaches.

## Sleeping Pills

Some medical doctors will prescribe sleeping pills to help with insomnia. Zopiclone is a common medication for insomnia but can have serious dependency if taken long-term.

# CHAPTER 15

# MENSTRUAL IRREGULARITIES

## Absent Menstrual Period – Amenorrhea

Amenorrhea is the absence of menstrual bleeding. It is normal when pregnant, before puberty or during menopause but if menses stops suddenly during the reproductive years, medical testing and investigation is warranted. Amenorrhea is classified into two categories: Primary and Secondary.

Primary Amenorrhea is when menstruation fails to occur by expected onset (usually by age 16).

Secondary Amenorrhea is when menstruation has previously occurred but has been absent for at least three months in a woman with a history of regular cycles or for six months in a woman with a history of irregular periods.

It has been estimated that the incidence of amenorrhea amongst women in the United States during their reproductive years is 1.8 to 3%. The prevalence in college-aged women is 2.6 to 5%. It may be seen in 20% of infertility cases.

### CAUSES

Complementary medicine usually won't be of any benefit if primary amenorrhea is due to a genetic or structural abnormality. If the cause is hormonal, complementary medicine may be helpful in most cases.

Primary Amenorrhea causes:

- Genetic abnormality (30% of cases) resulting in a defect or poorly formed genital or pelvic organs (missing uterus or vagina)
- Hormones play a large role in a woman's menstrual cycle. Hormonal imbalances/dysfunction in one or more of the following are usually a factor: the hypothalamus, pituitary, ovaries, adrenal glands and thyroid.
- Malnutrition – Anorexia nervosa
- Strenuous exercise – competitive athletes
- Radiation or chemotherapy exposure
- Infectious diseases that occur in the womb or after birth
- Pituitary tumours
- Autoimmune disease.

Secondary Amenorrhea causes:

*Women who are pregnant, breastfeeding, or in menopause are not considered to have Secondary Amenorrhea.*

- Toxin or radiation exposure
- Autoimmune disease
- Anemia (low iron or B12)
- Anorexia
- Obesity
- Strenuous exercise
- Nutritional deficiencies – Malabsorption/malnourished
- STRESS!
- Psychological factors
- Hypothalamus-Pituitary dysfunction
- Adrenal tumour
- Pituitary tumour or dysfunction (Sheehan's Syndrome)
- Low thyroid
- Elevated prolactin from the pituitary gland
- Polycystic ovaries or another ovarian dysfunction creating a lack of ovulation thus low progesterone levels
- Also, procedures such as a dilation and curettage (D and C) can lead

to scar tissue formation that may cause a woman to stop menstruating (Asherman's Syndrome). Scarring may also be caused by some severe pelvic infections.

## TESTING AND DIAGNOSIS

Some of the tests that will help determine the cause of primary or secondary amenorrhea include:

- Medical history, physical exam, breast exam, pelvic exam
- Pregnancy test
- Pelvic ultrasound to rule out polycystic ovaries
- Blood tests for estradiol, progesterone, testosterone, androstenedione, DHEA, cortisol, follicle stimulating hormone (FSH), Luteinizing hormone (LH), prolactin, thyroid function (TSH, T3, T4, rT3, thyroid antibodies) and insulin
- Genetic testing if necessary for Primary Amenorrhea
- CT or MRI to rule out pituitary or adrenal tumours
- Cholesterol panel.

## THERAPEUTIC CONSIDERATIONS

The first step at determining the cause of amenorrhea is usually done by a medical or naturopathic doctor using the tests above. Quite often, extreme fad dieting or eating disorders will lead to amenorrhea because of insufficient calories, too low dietary fat and low cholesterol. Don't forget that cholesterol is the backbone to all of the female hormones. If there is not enough cholesterol in the diet then the body does not have enough to make LH, FSH, estrogen, progesterone, testosterone, etc. High-level athletes, as well as health conscious individuals who engage in strenuous exercise, may experience an absence in menstruation from low body fat. Exercise-induced amenorrhea is very common among young women.

Due to the complexity of amenorrhea, it is impossible to address every cause in this chapter. Some of the causes such as tumours, systemic diseases and genetic disorders are beyond the scope of this book. We will, however, take an in-depth look at polycystic ovarian syndrome, thyroid disease and adrenal fatigue in the chapters to come. The key point to remember - always identify the cause before treating.

## PREVENTION and TREATMENT - Dietary and Lifestyle

## FOOD FACTORS

Both weight loss and obesity can be associated with amenorrhea. As mentioned above, extreme dieting, malnutrition and anorexia can all contribute to rapid weight loss and thus the lack of essential nutrients to support a healthy menstrual cycle. A whole food, nutrient-rich diet should be encouraged, focussing on the following:

- Adequate protein (at least 40 grams) in the forms of hormone and antibiotic-free animal proteins (chicken, turkey, lamb), fresh fish, legumes, organic soy products, eggs, nuts and seeds. Hormone and antibiotic-free red meat may be consumed one to two times a week.
- At least 1500 calories should be consumed daily, focussing on good fats. Underweight women with too little fat may result in low cholesterol and the inability to produce many hormones necessary for a normal menstrual cycle and ovulation. Healthy fats derived from olive oil, avocado, nuts and seeds, flaxseed and fish oil as well as organic dairy products should make up 20% of the caloric intake.
- Complex carbohydrates such as brown rice, millet, quinoa, oats, barley, buckwheat, amaranth and spelt should be consumed.
- As with the majority of health conditions, a diet low in refined and processed foods must be a priority.

## LIFESTYLE TIPS
- Maintain a healthy weight. Rapid weight gain or loss can adversely affect hormone levels and affect the hypothalamus from releasing hormones that regulate the menstrual cycle.
- Establish a good sleep schedule to help normalize hormones and proper ultradian rhythms (recurrent cycles repeated throughout a 24-hour circadian day).

- Assess for heavy metal toxicity. Do a gentle cleanse once a year.
- Maintain low stress levels, as chronic or high stress will negatively affect the hypothalamus and increase prolactin levels.
- Address any eating disorders with a health care team (medical doctor, naturopathic doctor, counselor, psychologist or others) to help monitor diet, eating patterns, exercise and address emotional issues and beliefs.

## KEY SUPPLEMENTS

### Calcium citrate or malate

A common cause of amenorrhea is premature ovarian failure in which there is a lower production of estrogen - as in menopause. These women are at risk of developing a lower bone density and increased risk for osteoporosis later in life. There is typically a decrease in calcium absorption in estrogen-deficient women.

DOSAGE: *1200 mg daily in divided doses*

### Magnesium bisglycinate or citrate

Magnesium is necessary for proper bone health. It supports healthy liver function, vitamin B6 and essential fatty acid metabolism.

DOSAGE: *600 mg daily in divided doses*

### Vitamin D3

Vitamin D is also necessary for proper bone health and supports a healthy immune system.

DOSAGE: *1000 IU daily*

### Vitamin B6

Vitamin B6 helps with proper hormone metabolism and liver function and is necessary for progesterone production.

DOSAGE: *100–200 mg daily*

## Flaxseed Oil and/or Pure Fish Oil (Omega-3 Fatty Acids)

Essential fatty acids in the form of flaxseed or uncontaminated fish oil block the formation of PGE2, which is a messenger molecule that promotes inflammatory pathways in the body. For amenorrheic women, fish and flaxseed oil are good fats that can help support healthy hormone production and balance.

DOSAGE: *Take up to 2 Tbsp of flax oil daily and/or up to 3000 mg fish oil daily with a minimum of 800 mg EPA and 400 mg DHA.*

## Chaste Tree Berry - *Vitex agnus castus*

Chaste Tree Berry (Vitex) is one of the single most important herbs for hormonal imbalances in women. The effect of chaste tree is on the hypothalamus/hypophysis axis in which it increases luteinizing hormone and has an effect that favours progesterone. Chaste tree can also stimulate ovulation which in turn will produce progesterone as well. Chaste tree may also inhibit prolactin release in the pituitary glands and be useful for those women who have no menstrual period due to elevated prolactin levels.

DOSAGE: *Take up to 400 mg daily.*
*It may take up to three months to see results.*

## Maca – *Lepidium meyeii*

Maca is a root vegetable cultivated in the Peruvian Andes that belongs to the brassica family. Maca is rich in amino acids, iodine, iron, and magnesium. Historically, Maca root has been used for its fertility- and libido-enhancing properties, as well as hormonal balancing effects.

A small study, treating women with premature ovarian failure with Maca for eight months, showed lower levels of follicle-stimulating hormone (FSH) and increased luteinizing hormone (LH). Elevated LH is necessary for ovulation and low FSH means that estrogen is being produced from the ovaries.

DOSAGE: *2–4 capsules daily of* **Ultimate Maca Energy**™, *1 tsp daily of* **MacaPunch Platinum Liquid Extract**™ *or 1 tbsp of* **Ultimate Maca Energy**™ *Powder (at least 3000 mg daily)*

## Liver Support – *EstroSense*®

Optimal liver function is essential for healthy hormone balance. Herbs such as calcium-d-glucarate, indole-3-carbinol, DIM and milk thistle help detoxify excess estrogens through the liver maintaining a healthy progesterone to estrogen ratio.

DOSAGE: *3 capsules twice daily*

## Adrenal Support – *AdrenaSense*®

Chronic stress and high cortisol levels affect the healthy balance of hormones and therefore, adrenal function should be addressed in those women with suspected adrenal fatigue. High cortisol levels raise prolactin levels.

DOSAGE: *1 capsule one to three times daily*

## Thyroid Support – *ThyroSense*®

Low thyroid disease is a common cause of amenorrhea. Thyroid function should be assessed with appropriate testing and supported if low. Many women with hypothyroidism and no menstrual cycle that are treated with thyroid support often have a return of a normal menstrual cycle.

DOSAGE: *2 capsules twice daily*

## CONVENTIONAL TREATMENT

### Hormone Replacement Therapy

If blood or saliva tests have confirmed that your amenorrhea is due to a hormonal imbalance and the above dietary and nutritional supplements have not brought on a period after three to six months, then a licensed medical or naturopathic doctor may prescribe hormone replacement therapy. Depending on the cause, each woman is assessed on an individual basis with dosing and timing of hormones prescribed accordingly.

## Heavy Periods – Menorrhagia

Excessive menstrual bleeding (menorrhagia) is a common complaint affecting 10-15% of women and becomes more common as women approach menopause. Menorrhagia often refers to a blood loss greater than 80 ml or 5 Tbsp, occurring during a regular menstrual cycle. It can involve excessive flow combined with prolonged bleeding.

Some women will describe:
- Soaking through one or more sanitary pads or tampons every hour for several consecutive hours
- Needing to use double sanitary protection to control the menstrual flow
- Needing to wake up to change sanitary protection during the night
- Bleeding for a week or longer
- Passing large blood clots with menstrual cycle
- Restricting daily activities due to heavy menstrual flow
- Symptoms of iron deficiency such as tiredness, fatigue or shortness of breath.

## CAUSES

Finding the root cause of the excessive flow is key, as with any disease. One theory proposed is a disturbance in prostaglandin production. Remember, prostaglandins are hormone-like molecules that are manufactured from fatty acids. Women who have heavy periods often have an abnormality in the biochemistry of the lining of the uterus (endometrium) in that they concentrate arachidonic acid to a much greater extent. Increased levels of arachidonic acid will increase the production of series 2 prostaglandins that are thought to be a major factor in both excessive bleeding and in menstrual cramping. Increased levels of arachidonic acid and series 2 prostaglandins drive inflammatory processes in the body.

Some other causes may include:

- Increased arachidonic acid in the lining of the uterus (endometrium) causing endometrium thickening and excess bleeding
- A hormonal imbalance that prevents ovulation. With no progesterone being produced, the result is excess bleeding. This can be triggered by stress, an infection, a neurotransmitter imbalance, being underweight, shift work, smoking and age.
- Vitamin A deficiency
- Food sensitivities/intolerances
- Excess toxicity, the need for detoxification
- Chronic illness or overexertion
- Iron deficiency
- Uterine fibroids or polyps
- Uterine or cervical infection
- Pelvic inflammatory disease
- Intrauterine devices (IUD)
- Pregnancy complications – A single, heavy, late period may be due to a miscarriage. An ectopic pregnancy – implantation of a fertilized egg within the fallopian tube instead of the uterus may also cause menorrhagia.
- Hypothyroidism
- Endometriosis
- Inherited bleeding disorders such as von Willebrand's disease (a condition in which an important blood-clotting factor is deficient or impaired)
- Medications such as anti-inflammatory medications and anticoagulants can contribute to heavy or prolonged menstrual bleeding.

## TESTING

The following tests are helpful at determining the cause of excessive bleeding during a normal menstrual cycle:

- Thyroid panel and basal body temperature

- Complete blood count, iron panel including: serum iron, ferritin (stored iron) and total iron-binding capacity (TIBC)
- Pregnancy test
- Pelvic exam and ultrasound to rule out uterine fibroids or polyps, and to measure the thickness of the uterine lining
- Endometrial biopsy or a dilation and curettage (D&C)
- Testing for sexually transmitted diseases (STDs)
- Pap smear
- Testing for clotting factors, prothrombin time
- Hormone testing of FSH, LH, estradiol, progesterone
- Serum vitamin A levels
- Food sensitivity testing.

**FACT - Did You Know?**

Research shows that 20% of teenage girls with heavy periods have a blood clotting disorder called von Willebrand's disease.

## PREVENTION and TREATMENT - Dietary and Lifestyle

## FOOD FACTORS

- Eat foods high in iron, especially when heavy periods persist on a monthly basis. Iron-rich foods include brewer's yeast, blackstrap molasses, organic red meat, eggs, dark leafy greens, apricots and legumes.
- It is important to include foods rich in vitamin K to help blood clotting and decrease heavy bleeding. These foods include dark leafy greens (kale, dandelion greens, collards, spinach, Swiss chard), scallions, Brussels sprouts, broccoli, asparagus and spices (cayenne, chili powder, paprika).
- Turmeric can be added to cooking, especially in curries, to decrease PGE2 (prostaglandins that promote inflammation).
- Emphasize consumption of fish high in omega-3s (salmon, herring, sardines, mackerel, anchovies) and reduce animal fats (beef, cheese, butter) and trans/hydrogenated fats to reduce arachidonic acid and

inflammatory pathways. Instead, promote anti-inflammatory healing pathways.

## LIFESTYLE TIPS

- Avoid xenoestrogens in the forms of plastics (BPA), phthalates in plastics and beauty products. Read labels carefully and avoid exposure to these hormone-mimicking compounds.
- Don't smoke!
- Do a gentle cleanse once a year, focussing on the bowels and liver.
- Avoid synthetic, bleached tampons that contain dioxin and other toxic chemicals.
- Exercise regularly to promote circulation and hormone metabolism. Brisk walking, jogging, swimming and biking are excellent aerobic activities. Don't forget to include weight resistance and core strengthening (yoga and pilates).
- Avoid or minimize coffee - it is inflammatory! Instead drink nettle (rich in iron), raspberry leaf (tonifies the uterus) or other naturally decaffeinated teas.

## KEY SUPPLEMENTS

### Vitamin K

Vitamin K may be helpful for women who experience heavy or prolonged periods. Increase green leafy vegetables as listed above or take in supplement form.

DOSAGE: *150–500 mcg daily*

### Vitamin A

A deficiency in vitamin A may contribute to heavy periods.

DOSAGE: *25,000 IU twice daily for acute bleeding or 10,000 IU daily for maintenance*

## Iron

Women who are iron-deficient are more likely to experience heavier menstrual cycles.

DOSAGE: *30–100 mg daily, depending on the severity of the anemia*
*Note: Do not take iron together with calcium since it will affect the proper absorption of each mineral.*

## Vitamin C and Bioflavonoids

Vitamin C and bioflavonoids help reduce heavy bleeding by strengthening the capillaries. In one study, vitamin C reduced heavy bleeding in 87% of the women. Vitamin C is also important for women who are iron-deficient as it helps increase iron absorption.

DOSAGE: *2000–4000 mg of vitamin C and 1000–2000 mg of bioflavonoids daily*

## Vitamin B Complex

One possible cause of heavy periods is estrogen dominance. The B vitamins help with metabolism of excess estrogen by supporting healthy liver function.

DOSAGE: *100 mg daily*

## Flaxseed Oil and/or Pure Fish Oil (Omega-3 Fatty Acids)

Essential fatty acids in the form of flaxseed or uncontaminated fish oil block the formation of PGE2, which is a messenger molecule that promotes inflammatory pathways in the body. Increased inflammation can cause heavy and prolonged menstrual bleeding.

DOSAGE: *Take up to 2 Tbsp of flax oil daily and/or up to 3000 mg fish oil daily with a minimum of 800 mg EPA and 400 mg DHA.*

### Chaste Tree Berry - *Vitex agnus castus*

Chaste Tree Berry (Vitex) is one of the single most important herbs for hormonal imbalances in women. The effect of chaste tree is on the hypothalamus/hypophysis axis in which it increases luteinizing hormone and has an effect that favours progesterone. This may be beneficial for estrogen-dominant conditions and thus help relieve symptoms of heavy bleeding and irregular cycles.

DOSAGE: *Take up to 400 mg daily.*
*\*It may take up to three months to see results.*

### Shepherd's Purse – *Capsella bursa-pastoris*

Shepherd's purse is a helpful herb for women with heavy menstrual cycles as it has the ability to coagulate blood. It is usually used in combination with other herbs such as Yarrow.

### Yarrow – *Achillea millefolium*

Yarrow is an astringent herb. These herbs are high in tannins and help draw together or constrict tissues or vessels making them very effective in stopping the flow of blood (heavy periods) or other secretions.

### Liver Support – *EstroSense®*

Optimal liver function is essential for healthy hormone balance. Herbs such as calcium-d-glucarate, indole-3-carbinol, sulforaphane, DIM and milk thistle help detoxify excess estrogens through the liver maintaining healthy progesterone to estrogen ratio. Anti-inflammatories and anti-oxidants such as curcumin, lycopene, rosemary extract and green tea extract are helpful in reducing inflammation.

DOSAGE: *3 capsules twice daily*

### Adrenal Support – *AdrenaSense®*

Chronic stress and high cortisol levels affect the healthy balance of hormones and therefore, adrenal function should be addressed in those women with suspected adrenal fatigue. Low adrenal function can also contribute to increased inflammation in the body and to increased PGE2 thus contributing to heavier periods.

DOSAGE: *1 capsule 1–3 times daily*

## Bio-identical Natural Progesterone Cream

Natural bio-identical progesterone cream may be used to correct infrequent periods, heavy periods or spotting in between periods.

DOSAGE: *¼–½ tsp twice daily, Day 15 to Day 26 (Day 1 is the first day of your menstrual cycle)*

## CONVENTIONAL TREATMENT

### Drug Therapy
- *Nonsteroidal anti-inflammatory drugs (NSAIDs).* NSAIDs such as ibuprofen (Advil, Motrin, others) or naproxen (Aleve), help reduce menstrual blood loss. NSAIDs have the added benefit of relieving painful menstrual cramps (dysmenorrhea).
- *Oral contraceptives.* Aside from providing effective birth control, oral contraceptives can help regulate menstrual cycles and reduce episodes of excessive or prolonged menstrual bleeding.
- *Oral progesterone.* When taken for ten or more days of each menstrual cycle, the hormone progesterone can help correct hormonal imbalance and reduce menorrhagia.
- *The hormonal IUD (Mirena).* This type of intrauterine device releases a type of progestin called levonorgestrel, which makes the uterine lining thin and decreases menstrual blood flow and cramping.

### Surgery
- *Dilation and curettage (D&C).* This procedure involves scraping or suctioning the tissue from the lining of the uterus to reduce menstrual bleeding. D&C procedures may have to be repeated if heavy bleeding persists.

- *Endometrial ablation.* This involves permanently destroying the entire lining of the uterus. After this procedure, most women will have little or no menstrual flow.
- *Hysterectomy.* This is the surgical removal of the uterus and cervix that results in the permanent cessation of menstruation and the inability to conceive.

## Menstrual Cramps – Dysmenorrhea

Dysmenorrhea is a common problem affecting over 50% of menstruating women of all ages. The term "dysmenorrhea" is derived from the Greek meaning "difficult monthly flow" thus referring to the pain experienced by women during their monthly cycle. Pain is often experienced just before or during the first two days of the menstrual period and will usually ease as the period continues. The pain can be in the pelvic region, lower back or may even radiate down the thighs. For some women, nausea, vomiting, fatigue, headache, increased urination and diarrhea may accompany the pain. It can be so debilitating that they are forced to take time off work or school, disrupting social and family life. It is estimated that 10% of women who experience menstrual cramps are rendered incapacitated for one to three days each month. Women with severe cases may even faint or experience dizziness. The symptoms can last from a few hours to one day but seldom longer than two to three days.

Dysmenorrhea can be classified as primary or secondary. In primary dysmenorrhea, the pain is monthly and associated with menstruation rather than a pelvic pathology or physical abnormality. Cramps usually arise within six to twelve months of the onset of menstruation, are more intense in women 20-24 years old and may decrease after childbirth. Smoking and being overweight are important risk factors for menstrual cramps. In contrast, secondary dysmenorrhea occurs when the menstrual pain is due to an underlying pelvic abnormality such as uterine fibroids, endometriosis, ovarian cysts, pelvic inflammatory disease, adhesions, polyps, congenital malformations or a narrowing of the cervical opening. Secondary dysmenorrhea may be present at the onset of menstruation but often develops later.

## CAUSES

There are a number of factors that play a role in contributing to menstrual pain and cramping:

- Increased levels of prostaglandins, specifically PGF2-alpha and PGE2 can cause uterine contractions and pain during menses. Prostaglandins are hormone-like compounds that are involved in hundreds of biochemical processes in the body. Studies have shown that women with menstrual cramps produce 8 to 13 times more PGF2-alpha than women without cramping or pain.
- Stress! Overwork or chronic illness.
- Pelvic or lumbar misalignment
- Poor circulation and therefore low oxygen delivery to the uterus
- Displacement of uterus. Some women will have their uterus displaced forward, backward or to the side thus making them more vulnerable to spasm.
- Liver and bowel toxicity. An imbalance of flora in the bowel or toxicity of the liver due to …TOO MUCH ESTROGEN. ☺

### PREVENTION and TREATMENT – Dietary and Lifestyle

A healthy diet is fundamental to treating women's menstrual cramps. Many women will experience relief from cramps simply by switching to healthier eating habits.

## FOOD FACTORS

- The most important foods to avoid are those that are high in arachidonic acid. Arachidonic acid is a fat that the body uses to produce prostaglandins PGE2 and PGF2-alpha – the ones responsible for increasing contractions in the uterus and increasing inflammation in the body. Fats found in red meat, dairy fat (butter, milk, cheese, yogurt, ice cream) and shellfish are the main sources of arachidonic acid promoting inflammation. Eliminating dairy products can have profound effects for as many as one third of women with menstrual cramps.

- Dairy products can also impair the absorption of magnesium. Magnesium is a key mineral responsible for many biochemical reactions in the body. It helps to reduce fluid retention, bloating and muscle cramping. Magnesium is found in Swiss chard, spinach, summer squash, pumpkin seeds and flaxseeds.
- Excess sugar and refined carbohydrates cause insulin to be secreted from the pancreas in high amounts. High insulin levels activate an enzyme called delta 5 desaturase. This enzyme will convert healthy fats such as borage oil, evening primrose, and vegetable oils into arachinonic acid thus promoting more inflammation in the body. If sugar is kept in check and thus insulin, this enzyme is not activated.
- While you might be drawn to these foods during a bout of PMS, avoid junk food, salty foods and high fatty and processed foods that promote water retention and inflammation.
- Too much sugar in the diet also interferes with the absorption and metabolism of some B vitamins and minerals. Deficiencies in some of these vitamins may worsen muscle tension and pain.
- Some of the best foods for decreasing menstrual cramps are those foods that promote anti-inflammatory prostaglandins, PGE1 and PGE3. Certain fish, such as salmon, halibut and sardines contain linolenic acid, a fat that helps relax muscles by producing the anti-inflammatory prostaglandins mentioned above. Some seeds and nuts are also sources of linolenic and linoleic acids and help to decrease inflammation. Flax, pumpkin, sesame and sunflower are excellent sources to add to salads or include in trail mix.
- Ensure at least 40 grams of fibre daily to promote healthy elimination from the bowels. Good fibre sources include flaxseeds, hemp hearts, oat bran, legumes, fruits and vegetables (see **Appendix**).

### FACT - Did You Know?

Ginger root (*Zingiber officinale*) has been found to have anti-inflammatory activity and has been used to treat menstrual cramping. In a double-blind trial, ginger powder (250 mg four times daily) was as effective as non-steroidal anti-inflammatory drugs for relieving pain in women with dysmenorrhea (menstrual cramps).

## LIFESTYLE TIPS

- Avoid caffeine in coffee, tea, chocolate and cola drinks.
- Avoid alcohol and other sources of sugar.
- Reduce salt consumption. Season foods with herbs and spices.
- Exercise at least 30 minutes most days to improve circulation, your general health, boost energy levels and lift your mood.
- See a bodyworker to manipulate and massage your lower back and reduce tension and stress in the body.
- Alleviate stress with exercise, yoga, meditation or massage.
- Use a nightly castor oil pack over the uterus the week before your period is due. *(*see **Appendix** *– Castor Oil Pack)*
- Reduce exposure to xenoestrogens in food and personal care products to minimize impact of endogenous estrogens. (see **Breast Cancer** Chapter)

## KEY SUPPLEMENTS

### Vitamin B6

Vitamin B6 (pyridoxal-5-phosphate) can be very helpful for the relief of PMS symptoms. It reduces some of the adverse effects of estrogen excess through supporting the liver's ability to metabolize more efficiently. Vitamin B6 is also needed to make beneficial prostaglandins to help reduce inflammation.

DOSAGE: *Take 50–100 mg/day with food, throughout the menstrual cycle. *Some women find that increasing the vitamin B6 dosage to 150–200 mg/ day during the week prior to menstruation enhances their response.*

### Curcumin

Curcumin is a potent antioxidant and is responsible for the yellow colour of turmeric. Curcumin is a powerful anti-inflammatory, decreasing the formation of inflammatory prostaglandins as well as helping with liver detoxification.

DOSAGE: *Take up to 500 mg, three times daily or 2 tsp of turmeric in food.*

## Flaxseed Oil and/or Pure Fish Oil

Essential fatty acids in the form of flaxseed or uncontaminated fish oil block the formation of PGE2, a messenger molecule that promotes inflammatory pathways in the body. Fish Oil is also very effective in controlling PMS food cravings.

DOSAGE: *Take up to 2 Tbsp of flax oil daily and/or up to 3000 mg fish oil daily with a minimum of 800 mg EPA and 400 mg DHA.*

## Calcium and Magnesium

Calcium and magnesium both have important roles in decreasing muscle spasms and pain in women experiencing menstrual cramps.

DOSAGE:

*Calcium citrate/malate – Take 800–1000 mg daily with food.*
*Magnesium bisglycinate/citrate – Take 300–500 mg daily with food.*

***All the above ingredients are found in **PMSense™**. It is an excellent product for relieving the symptoms of PMS, including menstrual cramping.

DOSAGE: *Take 2 capsules twice daily.*

## Vitamin C and Vitamin B3 (Niacin)

Combining vitamin C and niacin has shown promising results for women experiencing menstrual cramping. Some women however, will not enjoy the flushing effect of the niacin. Both the vasodilating effect from the niacin and an improvement in the permeability of the capillaries with the vitamin C, are thought to be the reason for the improvement in pain.

DOSAGE:
*Vitamin C – Take 500-1000 mg two times daily with food.*
*Vitamin B3 (Niacin) – Take 100 mg two times daily throughout the month and then every two to three hours during episodes of cramping.*

## Viburnum – *Viburnum opulus*
Crampbark is traditionally known for its anti-spasmodic and uterine tonifying effects. For these reasons, it is a commonly used herb for menstrual cramping and uterine or ovarian pain.

## Liver Support – *EstroSense®*
Increasing liver detoxification is vitally important to the elimination of harmful estrogens and improving all symptoms of PMS, including cramping and pain.

Important supplements such as milk thistle, curcumin, indole-3-carbinol, sulforaphane, calcium-d-glucarate, lycopene, milk thistle, rosemary extract and green tea extract help with the removal of excess harmful estrogens by metabolizing them through the liver.

DOSAGE: *3 capsules twice daily*

## Bowel Support – Probiotics and Fibre
Support the bowels with good bacteria such as *acidophilus* and *bifidobacterium*. Supplement with good fibre sources to help reduce bowel toxicity and improve healthy elimination.

*Ultimate Probiotic™ – One capsule twice daily with food.*
*FibreLean™ – One scoop twice daily in water, added to a smoothie or oatmeal.*

## CONVENTIONAL MEDICINE

## NSAIDS
Most medical doctors will often prescribe NSAIDS (non-steroidal

anti-inflammatory drugs) to be taken before the onset of a woman's menstrual period. Medications such as Advil, Motrin and Anaprox will block the formation of series 2 prostaglandins responsible for increasing pain and inflammation. Although these medications help to reduce the pain, they do not address the root cause. They are simply a "band-aid".

## Birth Control Pills

Birth control pills suppress ovulation and thus the hormonal changes of the menstrual cycle. Some women will experience a significant reduction in pain but the pills do cause havoc to normal hormone patterns if used long term.

―――――――――――― CHAPTER 16 ――――――――――――

# OSTEOPOROSIS

Osteoporosis is a degenerative disease involving the slow degradation of bone mass and integrity. The term osteoporosis is derived from the Greek *osteo* (bone) and *poros* (porous or passage) and refers to low bone mass and bone weakening. When bone is broken down faster than it can be rebuilt, it leads to increased bone fragility and the risk of fracture, particularly of the hip, spine and wrist. Osteoporosis is often referred to as a "silent disease" because it develops slowly over many decades. In fact, many people don't even discover they have osteoporosis until they break a bone or crack a rib.

Osteoporosis affects approximately 1.4 million Canadians, mainly postmenopausal women and the elderly. By the age of 50, the average Canadian woman has a 40% chance of suffering at least one fracture caused by brittle bones. One in every four Canadian women and one in every eight men over this age will be diagnosed with osteoporosis. Almost 30,000 hip fractures occur each year and this number is expected to quadruple by the year 2030.

If we look at the progression of bone growth throughout our lifetime, bones will steadily grow in length and density until the late teens. After this time, bones continue to increase in density but at a slower rate. Then, when you reach your 20s, bones achieve what's called "peak mass". This means that they stop building density and natural bone loss begins. Before menopause, women lose bone at a rate comparable to men (at a rate of one per cent per year). But with the loss of estrogen at menopause, women will lose bone two to six times faster. The rate of bone loss returns to one percent per year ten years after menopause.

## Bone Building Basics

Bone is living tissue that is constantly being broken down and rebuilt. Bone metabolism involves the removal of old bone from the skeletal system (bone resorption) and the addition of new bone (ossification). This process controls the healing and remodeling of bone during growth and following injuries such as fractures and micro-damage, which can occur during normal activity. In the first year of life, almost 100% of bone is replaced. In adults, remodeling proceeds at a rate of about 10% per year. The cells responsible for creating new bone are called osteoblasts and osteoclasts are the cells that break bone down. The structure of bone requires a close relationship and depends on the cooperation between these two cells. Adequate levels of calcium and other minerals as well as complex signalling pathways help achieve proper rates of growth. These signalling pathways include the action of several hormones, including the parathyroid hormone (PTH), vitamin D, growth hormone, steroids and calcitonin.

## Risk Factors

- Family history of osteoporosis
- Gastric or small-bowel resection, celiac or Crohn's disease (low absorption and assimilation of calcium)
- Sedentary lifestyle
- Heavy alcohol and tobacco use
- Hyperparathyroidism
- Hyperthyroidism or excess thyroid hormone medication
- Postmenopause
- Early menopause (physiological, surgical or drug-induced)
- Low calcium intake from diet
- Eating disorders (anorexia/bulimia)

- Long-term use corticosteroid therapy (prednisone or cortisone), chemotherapy or aromatase inhibitors to treat breast cancer, Depo-Provera injections, the antidepressant medications called selective serotonin reuptake inhibitors (SSRIs), methotrexate, heparin, some anti-seizure medications, the acid-blocking drugs called proton pump inhibitors and aluminum-containing antacids are all associated with an increased risk of osteoporosis.
- Nulliparity (never having been pregnant)
- Short stature and small bones
- Caucasian or Asian race
- High protein diet
- Excessive coffee or caffeinated beverages consumed daily
- Excessive soft drinks consumed daily
- Heavy metal toxicity
- Stress!

## SIGNS and SYMPTOMS

As mentioned above, osteoporosis is referred to as a "silent disease" because there are often no symptoms until one fractures a bone. There are, however, some warning signs that may indicate decreased bone density to help prevent fractures and worsening of bone loss. These include:

- Compression or stress fractures
- Gum disease or tooth decay
- Premature graying of hair (50% gray by age 40)
- Arthritis
- Low back pain
- Leg cramps at night
- Poor nail growth or brittle nails
- Decreased height.

## TESTS and DIAGNOSIS

Osteoporosis is best diagnosed using dual energy X-ray absorptiometry (DEXA). DEXA is considered the "gold standard" because it exposes a person to considerably less radiation than other x-ray procedures. In the DEXA scan, measurements of both the hip and lumbar spine are taken. A baseline at age 50 should be encouraged with re-tests done every two to four years. If any of the above risk factors apply, especially tobacco use, chemotherapy for breast cancer, amenorrhea (no period), Depo-Provera injections, menopause before age 45 or a history of fractures, start getting DEXA scans earlier.

## PREVENTION and TREATMENT – Dietary and Lifestyle

### FOOD FACTORS

To paraphrase a cliché, you are not simply what you eat, but also what you absorb. You can eat the world's best diet – replete with adequate fruits, vegetables, lean protein and whole grains – but if you can't absorb the nutrients, the food hasn't served you well. And the truth is, as we age, stomach acid becomes less effective. This leads to the inability to absorb some nutrients, including calcium. Be sure to eat plenty of raw fruits and vegetables so that you can benefit from the enzymes they contain. Remember that enzymes help us digest our food, but over-cooking destroys them. Enjoy your calcium in broccoli, collard greens, almonds, kale, sesame seeds and organic tofu (see **Calcium Content of Selected Foods** chart below*).*

When buying calcium supplements, avoid calcium carbonate as it is the most difficult to absorb. Choose calcium citrate or malate instead. Along with calcium, include magnesium in a 2:1 ratio of calcium to magnesium. Food sources of magnesium include kelp, millet, tofu, beet greens, swiss chard, buckwheat, brown rice, walnuts, pecans, and kidney beans.

Nowhere is the need for Vitamin D (in the form of cholecalciferol or Vitamin $D_3$) more obvious than when it comes to bone health. Vitamin $D_3$ increases calcium absorption by as much as 30 to 80%. Of course, our skin makes this vitamin in response to sunlight, but in Canada we simply don't have the climate to provide adequate sun exposure. You can get small amounts of Vitamin $D_3$ in egg yolks and fish oils but supplementing with Vitamin D$_3$ is recommended for optimal health.

## Calcium Content of Selected Foods

| Food | Mg per 3$^{1/2}$-oz serving |
|---|---|
| Kelp | 1,093 |
| Dulse | 298 |
| Collard greens | 250 |
| Kale | 249 |
| Turnip greens | 246 |
| Almonds | 234 |
| Parsley | 203 |
| Dandelion greens | 187 |
| Brazil nuts | 186 |
| Watercress | 151 |
| Goat's milk | 129 |
| Tofu | 128 |
| Figs, dried | 126 |
| Sunflower seeds | 120 |
| Yogurt | 120 |
| Sesame seeds | 110 |
| Broccoli | 103 |
| English walnuts | 99 |
| Soybeans, cooked | 73 |
| Pecans | 72 |
| Apricots, dried | 67 |
| Black currants | 60 |
| Dates | 59 |
| Prunes, dried | 51 |
| Pumpkin/squash seeds | 51 |
| Orange | 41 |
| Celery | 41 |
| Carrot | 37 |
| Sweet potato | 32 |
| Brown rice | 32 |

**FACT – Did You Know?**

Milk and dairy products are often promoted as a food that is good for the bones and prevents osteoporosis because of high calcium content. However, some studies have shown conflicting results between milk consumption and healthy bones. A 12-year prospective study of 77,761 female health professionals found that the incidence of hip fractures was not-significantly different in women who consumed two or more glasses of milk per day than in those who consumed one glass or less per week.

An observation reported by many complementary health care practitioners is that many of their patients have unrecognized allergies to milk protein. This chronic consumption of dairy may cause intestinal inflammation, potentially leading to malabsorption diseases and nutritional deficiencies that would negatively affect bone health.

Studies have shown that excess animal protein in the diet may promote bone loss. This can cause an increase in calcium being excreted through the urine. Certain animal protein such as red meat and pork can also acidify the blood causing calcium and other minerals to be leached from the bones to buffer the acidity. Healthy protein sources should include chicken, turkey, fish, legumes, organic soy products, nuts and seeds and eggs. Hormone and antibiotic-free lean animal meats should be encouraged.

High phosphorus in the diet is also implicated in osteoporosis. Phosphorus is usually found in carbonated drinks, including soft drinks. Drinking soft drinks daily reduces levels of calcium in the blood and therefore, the amount that can be deposited to the bones.

Other nutritional factors that speed up calcium loss from the bones and contribute to osteoporosis include:

- High salt
- Refined sugars
- Refined grains
- Caffeine in coffee, black tea and chocolate
- Alcohol.

Sticking to a more alkaline diet by reducing the above foods, including animal proteins (notably beef and pork), will help prevent osteoporosis as well. It has been theorized that the acidity from these foods causes minerals including calcium to be leached from the bones to buffer the blood. Alkaline foods, such as fruits and vegetables, will help with the buffering too and thus can prevent calcium loss from bone.

### FACT – Did You Know?

During periods of stress, the hormone cortisol is secreted from the adrenal glands. Cortisol inhibits the cells that form bone (osteoblasts). Thus, overproduction of cortisol results in the loss of bone density. For example, corticosteroids (such as prednisone) mimic the action of cortisol and will have the same effect on bone health. These drugs also decrease the amount of calcium that is absorbed from food and increase the amount of calcium lost in the urine.

## LIFESTYLE TIPS

- Get moving! Weight-bearing exercises stimulate osteoblasts (bone builders) to deposit in stressed areas of the bone as well as increase the secretion of calcitonin, a thyroid hormone that inhibits osteoclasts (bone breakers). An exercise program for bone building should include weight-bearing activities (jogging, walking, stair-climbing) at least 40 to 60 minutes daily and strength-training activities (weight-training, yoga or pilates) at least three times weekly.
- Avoid soft drinks! Phosphates in sodas bind with calcium from bones and both are excreted in urine.
- Avoid antacids! They lower the acid in your stomach and inhibit the absorption of calcium.
- Don't smoke!
- Avoid excessive consumption of alcohol.
- Drink at least 1 to 2 litres of filtered water daily. The neutral pH of the water will help keep the body more alkaline by flushing excess acids. You will be more acidic if you are dehydrated.
- Manage stress levels by practicing yoga, meditation and deep breathing exercises.

- Try to consume herbs or teas with high mineral content such as nettles, oatstraw, red raspberry leaves, chamomile, horsetail and dandelion greens.
- Check heavy metals! Cadmium and lead can be stored in bone and increase bone breakdown promoting osteoporosis. The most accurate method of testing is through the urine and can be done by a naturopathic doctor or complementary health care provider.

**FACT – Did You Know?**

How well the digestive system is working will determine how much calcium is absorbed. As we age, the level of stomach acid is greatly reduced. This has a big impact on how much calcium is absorbed and assimilated in the body. Studies have shown that 40% of postmenopausal women are severely deficient in stomach acid.

## KEY SUPPLEMENTS

### Calcium

Calcium is a key component for the prevention of osteoporosis as well as maintenance of good bone health. However, it must be remembered that calcium alone may only have a slight protective effect for bone health and that a combination of key bone builders, (*as discussed below*) is fundamental in any healthy bone program. The requirements for calcium increase as women age because of reduced intestinal calcium absorption due to low stomach acid. In the Women's Health Initiative (WHI) trial, hip fractures were significantly reduced in older women on calcium supplementation. The National Institutes of Health (NIH) recommends the following:

> **Body/Mind Connection**
> Osteoporosis is linked with feelings of having inadequate support. Realize and appreciate that life supports you in unexpected ways.

Premenopausal women aged 25-30
DOSAGE: *1000 mg/day*

Postmenopausal women under 65 using estrogen therapy
DOSAGE: *1000 mg/day*

Postmenopausal women not using estrogen therapy
DOSAGE: *1500 mg/day*

All women aged 65 and older
DOSAGE: *1500 mg/day*

There is a great deal of confusion and controversy about what form of calcium is the best. Oyster shell or bone meal calcium is often discouraged because of lead content. The most absorbable forms are often chelates that are bound to citrate, fumarate or malate. Calcium carbonate seems to be the least absorbable form.

It is also important to outline dietary calcium before deciding on how much calcium is needed in supplement form. Check out the calcium content of foods that you are consuming on a daily basis before taking large amounts of calcium supplements. You may be getting enough from diet alone!

DOSAGE: *1000–1500 mg daily in divided doses.*
***Note: Calcium supplements should be taken away from thyroid supplements or medications, zinc or iron.*

## Magnesium

When it comes to strong bones, magnesium supplementation may turn out to be as important as calcium supplementation. Magnesium regulates the parathyroid hormone and is necessary for the absorption of vitamin D. It is also involved in bone mineralization, with magnesium deficiency leading to the cessation of bone growth, decreased osteoblastic and osteoclastic activity, osteopenia (early bone loss) and bone fragility. Magnesium intake should be one half to three quarters of calcium intake.

DOSAGE: *500–750 mg daily of magnesium citrate or bisglycinate*

## Vitamin D3

Vitamin D is well known for its role in building strong bones and teeth as it promotes calcium absorption and utilization in the body. Vitamin D deficiency is quite common among women with osteoporosis. Vitamin D has proven to be useful for the reduction of fractures and the maintenance of bone health. A meta-analysis of five double-blind trials (including a total of 9,292 individuals at least 60 years of age) found that supplementation with 700-800 IU/day of Vitamin D reduced the incidence of hip fractures by 26%.

DOSAGE: *1000–4000 IU daily*

## Zinc

Zinc is an important mineral for bone formation by helping to form collagen in the bone matrix. It is required for the production of both osteoblasts and osteoclasts and improves the actions of Vitamin D.

DOSAGE: *15–30 mg daily*

## Copper

Copper plays a role in the cross-linking and stabilization of collagen in the bone matrix and in osteoblastic activity.

DOSAGE: *1–3 mg daily*

## Vitamin C

Vitamin C is an important antioxidant that plays an important role in collagen formation thus supporting the bone matrix. It also helps to reduce the risk of bone fracture in smokers.

DOSAGE: *2000 mg daily or to bowel tolerance*

## Ipriflavone

Ipriflavone is a synthetic flavonoid derived from the soy isoflavone, daidzein. It has been shown to slow down osteoclastic activity (bone breakdown) and increase bone-building activity. Research has found that treatment with ipriflavone for one to two years slowed bone loss in women during the first several years after the onset of menopause.

DOSAGE: *200 mg three times daily*
*\*Note: although rare, some women develop low white blood cell count while taking ipriflavone and therefore have your white blood cell count and lymphocytes checked before and every six months while taking ipriflavone.*

\*\*\*All the above nutrients are found in **OsteoSense Plus™** in combination with iodine, quercetin, boswelia, turmeric and broccoli sprout powder. This is an excellent formula to help promote bone formation, increase deposit of calcium into bone, promote proper absorption of calcium and help decrease acute and chronic osteoporosis and osteoarthritis pain.

DOSAGE: *2 capsules three times daily*

## Vitamin K2

Vitamin K is important for the maintenance of healthy bone. It is required for the production of osteocalcin, a protein found in large amounts in bone. Osteocalcin attracts calcium to bone tissue, enabling calcium crystal formation to occur and thus supporting bone mineralization. Vitamin K is an important component of bone formation and remodeling. Many studies have found that vitamin K levels were significantly lower in those patients diagnosed with osteoporosis and that decreased vitamin K intake was associated with an increased incidence in hip fractures in both men and women.

DOSAGE: *100 mcg daily*

## Boron
Boron has been found in research studies to reduce urinary excretion of calcium by 44%. It can also reduce urinary magnesium excretion and increase serum 17 beta-estradiol and testosterone levels.

DOSAGE: *3 mg daily*

## Strontium
Strontium is a trace mineral that is starting to gain more recognition for bone building. It supports the function of new bone growth while reducing the activity of bone breakdown and therefore increases bone mineral density.

DOSAGE: *700 mg daily to be taken one hour before breakfast or two hours after food, calcium supplements or milk products.*

## Silicon – *BioSil*™
Collagen is the most abundant protein found in the human body. It is a key structural protein involved in creating smooth skin, strong hair and nails and in supporting healthy flexible bones. Bone is actually made up of 30% collagen! The collagen in bone helps accumulate more calcium deposition through its calcium-binding sites. Therefore, increasing collagen increases calcium.

DOSAGE: *2 capsules daily or mix 6 drops in water or juice twice daily*

## Folic acid
Folic acid, vitamin B12 and B6 help breakdown high levels of homocysteine in the body. High homocysteine is associated with cardiovascular disease and an increased incidence of osteoporotic fractures. This may be due to the fact that high homocysteine damages collagen thus affecting the bone matrix and mineralization.

DOSAGE: *400–800 mcg daily*

## Vitamin B12

Vitamin B12 helps protect collagen from the damaging effects of high homocysteine in the body. Bone formation markers (osteoblast activity) such as alkaline phosphatase and osteocalcin are dependent on vitamin B12 status.

DOSAGE: *1000 mcg daily*

## Vitamin B6

Vitamin B6 also helps protect collagen from the damaging effects of high homocysteine in the body.

DOSAGE: *50-100 mg daily*

## Manganese

Manganese is required for bone mineralization and for the synthesis of connective tissue in cartilage and bone. Manganese stimulates the production of mucopolysaccharides so that calcification can take place.

DOSAGE: *15-30 mg daily*

## Flaxseed Oil and/or Pure Fish Oil

Essential fatty acids in the form of flaxseed or uncontaminated fish oil block the formation of PGE2, a messenger molecule that promotes inflammatory pathways in the body. Increased inflammation is associated with disrupting the acid/alkaline balance in the body. In order to buffer the acidity in the blood, calcium is leached from the bones. Elevated levels of PGE2 also correlate with increased urinary calcium excretion from the body. Reducing urinary calcium excreting would help prevent osteoporosis as well as reduce the formation of kidney stones. Essential fatty acids also help increase absorption of calcium in the body.

DOSAGE: *Take up to 2 Tbsp of flax oil daily and/or up to 3000 mg fish oil daily with a minimum of 800 mg EPA and 400 mg DHA.*

### Probiotics – *Lactobacillus acidophilus* and *Bifidobacterium* spp.

Probiotics are known to have an important role in the maintenance of normal flora in the gastrointestinal tract. They are involved in the absorption and assimilation of important vitamins and minerals. A healthy digestive tract with adequate "good" bacteria will help maintain bone health by assimilation of crucial bone-building nutrients.

DOSAGE: *at least 10 billion CFU daily with food*

### Adrenal Support – **AdrenaSense®**

As mentioned, high levels of cortisol during chronic stress inhibit the osteoblasts (bone builders) resulting in loss of bone density. Stress and high levels of cortisol create an acidic environment in the body. Vital bone-building minerals are forced from the bone to buffer the acidity in the blood. These minerals are then excreted in the urine.

DOSAGE: *Take 1–3 capsules daily with food.*

### Bio-Identical Estrogen and Progesterone

In some cases, a health care provider may prescribe bio-identical estrogen and progesterone for maintenance of bone health or for osteoporosis. Many studies have demonstrated that combinations of estrone, estradiol and estriol have a favourable effect on bone mineral density in postmenopausal women. Progesterone appears to promote bone formation by stimulating the osteoblasts (bone builders). Bio-identicals may not be suitable for everyone. Seek the guidance and advice from a complementary health care provider or naturopathic doctor to determine proper dosing and method of administration.

## CONVENTIONAL MEDICINE

- The most widely prescribed medications for osteoporosis are bisphosphonates. These drugs include: Alendronate (Fosomax), Risedronate (Actonel, Atelvia), Ibandronate (Boniva) and Zoledronic acid (Reclast, Zometa). Side effects include nausea, abdominal pain, difficulty swallowing and the risk of an inflamed esophagus or esophageal ulcers. Although rare, osteonecrosis of the jawbone can occur in some cases where a section of the jawbone dies and deteriorates.

- Raloxifene (Evista) mimics estrogen's beneficial effects on bone density in postmenopausal women. Hot flashes are a common side effect. This drug may increase the risk of developing blood clots.
- Calcitonin is a hormone produced by the thyroid gland that reduces bone resorption and may slow down bone loss. It is usually administered as a nasal spray and may cause nasal irritation in some individuals.

These medications reduce osteoclastic activity (bone breakdown) and increase mineralization of old bone tissue which, in some cases, will actually cause bones to become more brittle.

# PREMENSTRUAL SYNDROME - PMS

Premenstrual syndrome (PMS) is a complex of physical and psychological symptoms experienced by most women that occurs cyclically after ovulation, up to two weeks before the monthly menstrual period. The symptoms can vary from month to month in intensity but usually improve shortly after menstruation starts.

There are some 150 symptoms that have been assigned to PMS, most commonly:

- Low energy levels
- Anxiety
- Tension
- Irritability/anger
- Depression
- Headaches
- Breast tenderness
- Backache
- Abdominal bloating and swelling of the fingers and ankles.

It is estimated that 80% of menstruating women experience premenstrual emotional or physical changes with peak occurrences among women in their late 20s and early 30s. About 30% of women consider their PMS symptoms to be problematic, while 5 to 10% consider them debilitating and requiring medical intervention to manage their mood and behaviour changes. Some women with PMS experience premenstrual dysphoric disorder (PMDD). PMDD is a form of severe premenstrual syndrome associated with depression, hopelessness, anger, anxiety and low self-esteem.

## DIAGNOSIS

Diagnosing PMS is normally made by observation of symptoms, both mental and physical.

*Physical symptoms usually include:*
- Headaches/migraines
- Water retention
- Swelling of ankles, feet and hands
- Backache
- Abdominal cramps, heaviness or bloating
- Breast tenderness
- Weight gain
- Insomnia
- Acne
- Nausea, constipation or diarrhea.

*Mental symptoms include:*
- Food cravings
- Anxiety
- Panic attacks
- Poor concentration/memory
- Depression
- Irritability, hostility or aggressive behavior
- Fatigue
- Low sex drive
- Increased fears
- Low self-esteem or poor self image.

There has not been a consistent imbalance or deficiency identified to explain the complex array of physical and emotional symptoms that make up PMS. In the early 1980s, Guy Abraham, a leading researcher in the field, made an attempt to bring some order to the confusing picture. He proposed that PMS could be divided into four categories. Each was characterized by distinct symptoms related to their underlying cause and hormonal pattern. It is important to note that women generally fall into more than one category at once.

## PMS TYPES

PMS-A

PMS-A (ANXIETY) is the most common category and usually affects between 65 to 75% of PMS sufferers.
Common symptoms include:
- Anxiety
- Tension
- Irritability, anger
- Mood swings
- Insomnia
- Depression
- Suicidal thoughts
- Low self-esteem
- Sensitive to rejection or criticism
- Feeling overwhelmed.

Symptoms in this category are thought to be strongly associated with excessive estrogen and deficient progesterone levels in the latter half of the menstrual cycle (post-ovulatory or luteal phase). A drop in serotonin levels as well as thyroid and adrenal function can also impact moods and PMS-A symptoms.

PMS-H

PMS-H (HYPERHYDRATION or WATER RETENTION) is the second most common category, occurring in 60 to 66% of patients.

Common symptoms include:
- Breast swelling and tenderness
- Abdominal bloating
- Weight gain of over three pounds
- Swelling of the face, hands, fingers and ankles.

These symptoms are primarily due to an increase in body fluid volume from increased levels of the hormone aldosterone. Aldosterone is an adrenal hormone that is elevated during stress. Increased amounts of this hormone will cause water to be retained in the body. Increased levels of estrogen relative to progesterone, a magnesium deficiency as well as excess amounts of salt in the diet will all cause salt and water retention.

## PMS-C

PMS-C (CRAVINGS) typically affects 33% of PMS sufferers.
Common symptoms include:
- Cravings for sweets, carbohydrates and chocolate
- Increased appetite
- Headaches
- Fatigue
- Feeling faint, dizziness
- Heart palpitations.

An abnormal glucose tolerance test (GTT) is usually seen five to ten days before menses thus implying an excess secretion of insulin in response to increased sugar consumption. The GTT is usually normal during the rest of the menstrual cycle. Theories explaining the cravings for sugar include a drop in cortisol levels, low serotonin and a deficiency in PGE1 (a beneficial prostaglandin). Consumption of carbohydrates will increase brain uptake of tryptophan (precursor of serotonin) thereby increasing serotonin synthesis in the brain.

## PMS-D

PMS-D (DEPRESSION) affects 25 to 35% of PMS sufferers.
Common symptoms include:
- Depression

- Forgetfulness, clumsiness
- Confusion
- Lethargy, sluggishness, fatigue
- Withdrawal, disinterest in usual activities
- Insomnia.

A drop in thyroid hormones as well as low serotonin levels during the premenstrual phase may trigger symptoms.

Other causative theories for premenstrual syndrome include:

- Serotonin/tryptophan deficiency or excess
- Norepinephrine/tyrosine deficiency
- Hypothyroidism
- Androgen deficiency or excess
- GABA deficiency
- Essential fatty acid deficiency resulting in abnormal prostaglandin synthesis
- Magnesium deficiency
- Stress
- Dopamine deficiency
- Vitamin B6 deficiency.

It is highly probable that an imbalance, involving the interaction of hormones, nutrients and neurotransmitters combined with stress, will cause the symptoms of PMS. The imbalances may differ quite widely among women or even from cycle to cycle in the same woman. Some postulate that PMS may be an abnormality in the way a woman adapts to her monthly hormone fluctuations.

## THERAPEUTIC CONSIDERATIONS

### Estrogen Dominance and Liver Function

A basic foundation for many complementary health care practitioners in their approach for treating PMS is the concept of the liver's role in detoxification. The theory is that if liver function is compromised or "sluggish" then estrogen metabolism is diminished, leading to excess estrogen levels and thus an "estrogen-dominant" state.

Estrogen excess is known to produce cholestasis, which means diminished bile flow or stasis of bile. Bile is produced in the liver and stored in the gallbladder; it is responsible for the digestion of fats and assisting in the proper elimination of harmful estrogen metabolites. Cholestasis can also be caused by alcohol, anabolic steroids, excess estrogen including birth-control pills and hormone replacement, the presence of gallstones, hereditary disorders such as Gilbert's syndrome, pregnancy and various drugs (erythromycin and cimetidine). The presence of cholestasis leading to estrogen excess may be one of the factors contributing to PMS.

## Estrogen Dominance and Neurotransmitters

Estrogen excess can negatively impact neurotransmitter synthesis and endorphin activity. Neurotransmitters are chemical messengers released from nerve cells within the brain that transmit information to other cells in the body. For example, the neurotransmitter serotonin is a chemical messenger that has a role in modulating anxiety, mood, sleep, appetite and sexuality. A lower level of serotonin or dopamine is thought to be connected to mood and depression in PMS and for that reason, antidepressants are gaining popularity among many medical doctors for the treatment of PMS. Women should be aware that resorting to antidepressants is not their only option. Normalizing estrogen to progesterone ratios can help increase neurotransmitters such as serotonin, improving mood and overall well-being.

Endorphin levels may also be affected by estrogen dominance. Endorphins are chemical compounds that help with elevating mood and relieving pain. Low levels of endorphins have been found to be quite common among women with PMS. These levels are normally decreased by stress and raised by exercise. Supporting healthy adrenal function and increasing blood circulation with daily exercise is vitally important.

## Vitamin B6 Deficiency

Many studies have been reported on the use of vitamin B6 for the treatment of PMS as well as for women complaining of depression associated with oral contraception (oral contraception and HRT are known to deplete vitamin B6 levels in the body). An overview of these studies has been published in the *British Journal of Obstetrics and Gynaecology* showing substantial effects on a wide range of PMS symptoms. These impressive outcomes are thought to be due to the involvement of vitamin B6 in the synthesis of important neurotransmitters such as serotonin and dopamine. Lower levels of these brain neurotransmitters have been implicated in the symptoms of PMS. Vitamin B6 is also essential for proper estrogen detoxification. It has been postulated that a deficiency in vitamin B6 decreases estrogen detoxification by the liver and hence leads to estrogen dominance.

## Magnesium Deficiency

Some symptoms of magnesium deficiency can be very similar to PMS symptoms such as anxiety, depression, irritability and headaches. Studies have shown significantly lower plasma levels of magnesium in women with PMS symptoms versus those who do not experience PMS.

Magnesium may also be helpful in assisting vitamin B6 and essential fatty acid metabolism. One study found that the combination of magnesium and vitamin B6 improved PMS symptoms more effectively than each one on their own.

## Prostaglandin Imbalance

Prostaglandins are modified forms of unsaturated fatty acids that are synthesized in virtually all cells of the body and which act as chemical messengers. PMS could result from a disturbance in the body's production of prostaglandins and a consequent imbalance of the various female hormones. Excessive and incorrect prostaglandin (PG) synthesis has been implicated as a cause of PMS. Furthermore, a deficiency of prostaglandin E1 (PgE1) at the central nervous system has been proposed to be involved in PMS. There are many nutrients important for the synthesis of PgE1. These include magnesium, linoleic acid, vitamin B6, zinc, vitamin C and vitamin B3. This theory is carried through as a basis for some of the nutritional therapies in the treatment of PMS.

### Estrogen's Effect on Aldosterone and Prolactin

Aldosterone is a hormone produced by the adrenal glands that helps regulate sodium and potassium levels in the body. This helps control blood pressure and the balance of fluids and electrolytes in the body.

Many women with PMS will experience water retention prior to the onset of menses. This is often caused by excess estrogen leading to an increase in aldosterone levels and thus an increase in fluid retention.

An excess in prolactin can also been seen in many cases of PMS especially in women experiencing breast pain or fibrocystic breast disease. Prolactin is a hormone naturally released by the pituitary gland that stimulates breast development and milk production in women. Estrogens made both inside the body as well as from exogenous sources (e.g. man-made chemicals such as BPA), birth control pills or hormone replacement therapy are all known to increase prolactin secretion. High levels of prolactin can also cause infertility, anxiety, irritability, and other menstrual abnormalities such as PCOS.

 **FACT - Did You Know?**

Some practitioners have reported that an "anti-candida" program relieves PMS symptoms in some cases. With women who have a history of recurrent vaginal yeast infections or have been treated with antibiotics, oral contraceptives or systemic glucocorticoids, candida should definitely be considered as a causative factor.

## PREVENTION and TREATMENT – Dietary and Lifestyle

## FOOD FACTORS

- Sugar has several detrimental actions in PMS. Try to reduce or avoid sugars in the forms of high fructose corn syrup, white flour (cookies, pastries, white bread/rice/pasta), fruit juices with added sugar and colas. Read food labels carefully and avoid added sugars such as glucose, sucrose, fructose, and corn syrup.

- Consume at least three servings of organic fruits and six servings of organic vegetables daily.
- Increase whole grains (barley, brown rice, amaranth, quinoa, millet, buckwheat).
- Minimize dairy products such as milk, cheese and butter. Although dairy products do contain calcium, as we age they become increasingly more difficult to digest and can aggravate inflammation in the body, therefore contributing to symptoms of PMS. A small amount of plain, organic, low-fat yogurt or goat cheese in moderation is acceptable.
- Include free-range, hormone and antibiotic-free protein sources such as chicken, lamb and turkey and organic, non-GMO tofu, beans, nuts and seeds as protein sources.
- Some research has linked calcium to the reduction of physical and psychological symptoms of PMS. Be sure to get adequate calcium from collard greens, basil, cinnamon, kale, sesame seeds and asparagus.
- Vitamin E is helpful in reducing the production of prostaglandins involved with cramping and breast tenderness. Consume vitamin E in sunflower seeds, almonds, papaya, olives and blueberries.
- Adding garlic, tuna, bananas, carrots and cabbage to your menu will increase vitamin B6. This vitamin may also help ease PMS symptoms. Be sure to enjoy fresh B6 foods, as up to 60 or 80% of the nutrient is lost in the canning process and 15% is lost during freezing.

## LIFESTYLE TIPS

- A wellness journal will help you make connections between diet and lifestyle choices and your symptoms. Record foods you eat, mood, activities, sleep patterns, the commencement of symptoms, the beginning and end of your menstrual flow and when symptoms subside. Do this for at least two cycles or for as long as it takes to isolate your personal triggers.
- Due to the association of PMS with hypothyroid, be sure to have

your thyroid levels checked. (see **Hypothyroid** Chapter)

- Women with PMS should avoid caffeine especially if major symptoms include anxiety, depression, breast tenderness or fibrocystic breast disease. Replace caffeinated beverages with herbal or green tea.
- Avoid foods that contain PCBs, dioxins, BPA and heavy metals.
- Avoid alcohol or drink minimally (once per week).
- Drink at least two litres of pure, filtered water daily.
- Avoid animal-derived (saturated) fats and hydrogenated vegetable oils.
- Cook with extra-virgin olive oil on low heat and if cooking at high heat, use coconut oil.
- Avoid excess salt if you suffer from water retention during PMS.
- Several studies have shown that women who exercise regularly do not suffer from PMS as often as those women who lead a sedentary lifestyle. Engage in a regular exercise program with both cardiovascular and weight-bearing exercises.

## KEY SUPPLEMENTS

### Vitamin B6

Vitamin B6 (Pyridoxal-5-phosphate) can be very helpful for the relief of PMS symptoms. In addition to reducing some of the adverse effects of estrogen excess through supporting the liver's ability to metabolize more efficiently, Vitamin B6 may increase the concentrations of the neurotransmitters serotonin and dopamine as well as the hormone progesterone. Research has found that vitamin B6 can be helpful for relieving edema, bloating, headaches, breast pain, depression, irritability and possibly acne flare ups.

DOSAGE: *Take 50–200 mg/day with food, throughout or prior to the menstrual cycle.*
*\*Some women find that increasing the vitamin B6 dosage to 150–250 mg/ day during the week prior to menstruation enhances their response.*

## Magnesium – *Magnesium Bisglycinate*

Symptoms of magnesium deficiency can be very similar to some PMS symptoms such as anxiety, depression, irritability and headaches.

Some studies have shown significantly lower plasma levels of magnesium in women with PMS symptoms versus those who do not experience PMS.

Magnesium may also be helpful in assisting vitamin B6 and essential fatty acid metabolism. One study found that the combination of magnesium and vitamin B6 was more effective in improving symptoms of PMS than each one individually.

DOSAGE: *Take 200 mg one to three times per day with food.*

## Curcumin

Curcumin is a potent antioxidant and is responsible for the yellow colour of turmeric. Curcumin has numerous health benefits due to its powerful anti-inflammatory properties. It supports joint health, liver function and the gastrointestinal and cardiovascular systems. Curcumin also assists in the detoxification of harmful estrogens through the liver.

DOSAGE: *Take up to 500 mg, three times daily or 2 tsp of turmeric in food.*

## Flaxseed Oil and/or Pure Fish Oil (Omega-3 Fatty Acids)

Essential fatty acids in the form of flaxseed or uncontaminated fish oil block the formation of PGE2 which is a messenger molecule that promotes inflammatory pathways in the body. Fish Oil is also very effective in controlling PMS food cravings.

DOSAGE: *Take up to 2 Tbsp of flax oil daily and/or up to 3000 mg fish oil daily with a minimum of 800 mg EPA and 400 mg DHA.*

## Chaste Tree Berry - *Vitex agnus castus*

Chaste Tree Berry (*Vitex*) is one of the single most important herbs for relief of PMS symptoms. The effect of chaste tree is on the hypothalamus/hypophysis axis in which it increases luteinizing hormone and has an effect which favours progesterone. It has been shown to decrease prolactin levels, thought to be a factor in PMS.

DOSAGE: *Take up to 250 mg daily.*
*\*It may take up to three months to see results.*

\*\*\*All the above nutrients are found in **PMSense™**, an excellent formula for relieving the symptoms of PMS.

DOSAGE: *Take 2 capsules twice daily.*

## 5-HTP – **HappySense®**
5-HTP is the precursor to serotonin, our "happy hormone".
5-HTP in combination with vitamin B6 may improve PMS tension, mood swings, and irritability by increasing serotonin levels.

DOSAGE: *50mg/100mg Take 1 to 2 capsules three times daily.*

## St. John's Wort
St. John's Wort helps increase serotonin levels but should be avoided if you are taking any conventional anti-depressant.

DOSAGE: *Take 300 mg one to three times daily.*

## Thyroid Support – **ThyroSense®**
A low thyroid function (hypothyroidism) has been shown to contribute to PMS symptoms, especially with moods and depression.

DOSAGE: *Take 2 capsules twice daily.*

## Adrenal Support – **AdrenaSense®**
Supporting adrenal function will help to normalize cortisol and aldosterone levels and will decrease sugar cravings and water retention.

DOSAGE: *Take 1 to 3 capsules daily with food.*

## Liver Support – *EstroSense®*

Increasing liver detoxification is vitally important to the elimination of harmful estrogens and improving all symptoms of PMS.

Important supplements such as milk thistle, curcumin, indole-3-carbinol, sulforaphane, calcium-d-glucarate, DIM, green tea extract, lycopene and rosemary extract help support estrogen metabolism and bind harmful by-products promoting their elimination from the body.

DOSAGE: *3 capsules twice daily*

**FACT – Did You Know?**

A study reported in *Human Psychopharmacology* in 2003 found that chaste tree berry was as effective as the drug Prozac for PMS symptoms. Another study found a 51% improvement in PMS symptoms after two months of treatment with 300 mg St. John's wort.

## CONVENTIONAL MEDICINE

### Progesterone Cream

Progesterone is commonly prescribed for PMS by both conventional and complementary health care practitioners, usually after a progesterone deficiency has been identified. Progesterone levels should be monitored regularly by saliva or blood tests (every three to six months) and dosage adjusted accordingly.

A commonly prescribed progesterone is oral Prometrium (a micronized natural progesterone) available in capsule form (100 or 200 mg) or as a cream (containing approximately 400 mg of natural progesterone per ounce). Dosage and timing is dependent on symptoms and a woman's individual PMS history.

Some creams may not actually contain progesterone. Wild yam or soy-based creams might be ineffective because they have not been pharmaceutically converted into actual progesterone. It is best to contact a compounding pharmacy or have your MD or ND write up a prescription.

## Antidepressants – Selective Serotonin Reuptake Inhibitors (SSRIs)

Some women find taking Prozac (fluoxetine) and sertraline very effective in decreasing PMS symptoms when taken two weeks prior to their menstrual period. SSRIs prolong serotonin levels and activity in the brain and therefore, improve mood and irritability. Side effects include headaches and weight loss as well as a high incidence of orgasm dysfunction.

## Birth Control Pills

The pill is often used to minimize PMS symptoms by "normalizing" hormonal imbalances. Some women, however, find that their symptoms worsen. Also, when they decide to discontinue the birth control pill after years of use, it becomes much more difficult to regulate their cycle. The birth control pill depletes many important vitamins and minerals. Women who are taking the BCP should supplement accordingly. (see **Birth Control** Chapter)

*Remember...*
Conventional treatment should be a last resort. PMS symptoms can be easily resolved by addressing the root cause through lifestyle and diet support and effective nutritional and herbal supplementation.

# CHAPTER 18

# POLYCYSTIC OVARY SYNDROME - PCOS

Affecting between 6 and 10% of women, polycystic ovary syndrome (PCOS) is also known as Stein-Leventhal syndrome and polycystic ovarian disease. This hormonal disorder causes ovaries to produce higher than normal amounts of androgens (male hormones) which can interfere with egg production. Eggs normally produced by the ovaries develop into fluid-filled cysts. As a result, instead of releasing an egg during ovulation, the cysts become enlarged. Although PCOS originates in the ovaries, changes in hormone levels affect many body systems and can create long-term health consequences.

The most common characteristics of PCOS are obesity, hirsutism (excess hair growth on women in those parts of the body where hair does not normally occur) and problems with ovulation (irregular, infrequent or absent) which often lead to fertility problems. However, not all women have the above classic symptoms. In fact, less than 50% of women with PCOS are obese. Many of the women diagnosed with PCOS are of normal weight or even underweight, have no excess hair growth on the face or chest and may even have normal menstrual cycles.

## SIGNS and SYMPTOMS
PCOS signs and symptoms often begin soon after a woman first begins

having periods. In some cases, PCOS develops later on during the reproductive years. PCOS symptoms can vary from person to person, in both type and severity. Some common signs and symptoms include:

- Infrequent or absent menstrual periods
- Excessive bleeding during your period
- Skin tags, typically in the armpits or neck area
- Excess facial hair
- Scalp hair thinning
- Acne
- Weight gain, obesity (especially abdominal weight)
- Increased blood sugar
- High levels of cholesterol and triglycerides in the blood, low levels of HDL ("good" cholesterol) and high levels of LDL ("bad" cholesterol)
- Elevated cortisol
- Increased susceptibility to hypothyroidism
- Elevated insulin levels or insulin resistance
- Elevated LH (luteinizing hormone) which causes the ovaries to produce more androgens
- Elevated androstenedione and testosterone
- Infertility or subfertility
- Recurrent miscarriage
- High prolactin
- High levels of estrogen, especially estrone
- Low levels of sex hormone binding globulin (SHBG) inhibited by high levels of insulin. Therefore more estrogen and testosterone are circulating in the body.
- Enlarged ovaries with multiple small cysts in the ovary
- Skin hyper-pigmentation.

Untreated PCOS can lead to increased risk of:

- Infertility

- Excessive hair growth
- Type 2 diabetes and gestational diabetes
- Heart disease
- Bleeding in the uterus
- Increased risk of miscarriage
- Sleep apnea
- Uterine cancer
- Fibrocystic breast disease.

## CAUSES

Historically, PCOS was believed to be caused entirely by the surplus production of androgens but recent research shows that high insulin levels (hyperinsulinemia) and insulin resistance are key instigators. Insulin resistance means that cells don't respond effectively to insulin and sugar is denied entry to cells. Because having excess blood sugar is dangerous, in cyclical fashion, the pancreas responds by releasing more insulin.

Too much insulin causes the body to release extra androgens. In one study of teens with PCOS, almost 70% also had insulin resistance. Other research shows that PCOS patients with insulin resistance also tend to be more obese, have more upper body fat and more skin hyperpigmentation.

High levels of androgens and insulin resistance are known to disturb the production of female hormones, including luteinizing hormone (LH) and follicle-stimulating hormone (FSH), which control the menstrual cycle and ovulation. Obviously then, this leads to the irregular menstrual cycles and missed ovulation for women with PCOS.

PCOS seems to have a genetic component, and therefore can, but does not necessarily, run in families. Some research shows that excessive exposure to male hormones (androgens) in fetal life may permanently prevent normal genes from functioning properly. This may promote a male pattern of abdominal fat distribution which increases the risk of insulin resistance and low-grade inflammation.

Inflammation caused by poor diet, environmental toxins and stress can lead to insulin resistance and cholesterol accumulation in the blood vessels (atherosclerosis). Research has shown that women with PCOS have low-grade inflammation.

## TESTING and DIAGNOSIS

The diagnosis of PCOS is a difficult one because there is no one specific test to definitively diagnose it. Practitioners often rule out other disorders that may mimic symptoms of PCOS and diagnosis is often one of exclusion. The current diagnostic criteria from the 2003 Rotterdam PCOS consensus is that at least two of the following three features must exist:

- Chronic anovulation (lack of ovulation, irregular periods)
- Clinical (acne, excess hair, oily hair, thickened skin, male pattern balding) or biochemical signs of hyperandrogenism (elevated levels of male hormones or androgens)
- Polycystic ovaries on ultrasound.

Some important blood tests to assist with the diagnosis of PCOS:

- Free testosterone
- DHEA
- LH/FSH
- Prolactin
- TSH, T3, T4, anti-microsomal antibodies, anti-thyroglobulin antibodies
- HDL, LDL, triglycerides, cholesterol, c-reactive protein
- 17-hydroxyprogesterone
- Fasting insulin and glucose, glucose tolerance test.

## PREVENTION and TREATMENT – Dietary and Lifestyle

## FOOD FACTORS

Excess weight can be a major concern for those with PCOS. Aim to reduce weight through healthy lifestyle changes involving regular exercise and the blood sugar stabilizing low GI diet. Research supports following the low GI diet for women with PCOS (see **Appendix** - *Glycemic Index of Foods*). Avoiding high glycemic carbohydrates such as white rice, corn, millet and white flour will prevent blood sugar spikes throughout the day. Including complex carbohydrates such as barley, quinoa and legumes will help keep blood sugars stable and prevent insulin resistance. Soluble fibre will also help control insulin levels and promote the elimination of excess androgens through the bowel. Include apples, cabbage, raw carrots, oatmeal, oat bran, flaxseeds, psyllium and beans regularly in the diet.

It is important to instruct women to eat a well-balanced diet focusing on low GI foods and eating regularly. By eating five smaller meals throughout the day rather than eating three larger ones will help keep blood sugars balanced. It is also important to include healthy proteins such as lean hormone and antibiotic-free meats, nuts and seeds, legumes, organic tofu or tempeh, fish and eggs with each meal to avoid blood sugar spikes.

Sugar is also hidden in many processed and packaged foods as well as juices and sugary drinks. Avoid artificial sweeteners such as sucralose and aspartame and choose natural sugars - fruit, stevia or agave. Also drink PLENTY of pure filtered water and herbal tea.

There are several natural substances that bind to and stimulate sex hormone binding globulin (SHBG) which then binds some of the testosterone in the blood stream, which in turn reduces the hyperandrogenism of PCOS. SHBG will also bind excess estrogen to prevent estrogen dominance in some women. The root of the nettles plant contains many lignans and these compounds have an affinity to SHBG in humans.

Green tea has been shown to reduce excess testosterone levels and to control high levels of insulin. Drink green tea instead of caffeinated beverages such as coffee, tea, hot chocolate or colas.

Flax seeds and soy are two important foods relevant in a PCOS diet. Again, flax seeds contain lignans which increase SHBG. This results in a lowering of blood testosterone levels and perhaps reducing the hyperandrogenic effects. Add 2 Tbsp of ground flax meal to a smoothie, oatmeal or sprinkle on a salad.

Reduce your exposure to xenoestrogenic (estrogen-mimicking) chemicals in fertilizers, pesticides and herbicides by consuming organic produce as often as possible. Likewise, if you consume (low-fat) dairy and meat, choose the organic varieties to reduce your exposure to animal hormones.

 **FACT – Did You Know?**

There are many spices and herbs that can help support healthy insulin activity and blood sugar balance. Add cinnamon and nutmeg to oatmeal, cook up curry using turmeric or add bay leaves to a stew or soup.

## LIFESTYLE TIPS

- Because stress is a factor in increasing levels of androgens, employ strategies to reduce stress in your life. Support your adrenal glands. (see **Adrenal Fatigue** Chapter)
- Stress reduction may also help alleviate PCOS-related acne.
- Use a natural shampoo and conditioner. Avoid xenoestrogenic ingredients including phthalates and parabens in all of your personal care products. (see **Breast Cancer** Chapter)
- Some research links excess androgen exposure in young girls (from fetus to puberty) with increased risk of PCOS. Pregnant women and mothers should be vigilant about the exposure of their female children to androgens. Using natural health care products will be helpful.
- Although those with PCOS can experience difficulty maintaining healthy weight, reducing excess weight can help with symptom relief.
- Try to incorporate a regular exercise program including both weight resistance and aerobic activity. Exercising four to six hours a week will help increase muscle mass, burn fat more efficiently, balance hormones and help with healthy blood sugar and insulin levels.
- In women with PCOS, cigarette smoking increases free testosterone and fasting insulin levels, resulting in increased insulin resistance.

For symptom relief, do not smoke.

- Try acupuncture for relief of symptoms and hormone balancing.

## KEY SUPPLEMENTS

### Chromium picolinate or chelate

Chromium is one of the most researched nutritional interventions in the treatment of glucose and insulin imbalances. Chromium has been used in a number of studies on insulin resistance. In one study published in the *American Journal of Clinical Nutrition*, a dose of 200 mcg of chromium daily resulted in improvements in both glucose tolerance and circulating insulin levels. Further research investigated the use of chromium as a sole treatment for type 2 diabetes. When patients were given 100 or 500 mcg chromium twice daily both fasting and two-hour postprandial glucose levels significantly decreased for both chromium treatment groups.

> **Body/Mind Connection**
> Your ovaries are your creative centre. Focus on finding balance with your creative flow.

DOSAGE: *100–500 mcg in divided doses with food*

### Gymnema sylvestre

Gymnema has been researched predominantly for its antidiabetic actions and has shown promising results for both type 1 and type 2 diabetes. In a study of type 2 diabetics, 400 mg of Gymnema extract was administered daily to 22 patients over the course of 18 to 20 months. This was in addition to their oral hypoglycemic medications. Significant reductions in blood sugar and HbA1c were demonstrated as well as an increase in the release of insulin by the pancreas. Medication dosages were decreased and five people were able to discontinue drugs entirely.

DOSAGE: *400 mg daily*

## Fenugreek extract – *Trigonella foenum graecum*

Fenugreek has been used as a remedy for diabetes, particularly in India. Administration of defatted fenugreek seed powder has been shown to reduce blood levels of glucose, insulin, total cholesterol and triglycerides, and increase HDL cholesterol levels.

DOSAGE: *50 mg twice daily*

## Bitter Melon – *Momordica charantia*

Bitter melon has been used extensively in folk medicines as a remedy for diabetes.

DOSAGE: *100–200 mg three times daily*

## Alpha-lipoic Acid

Alpha-lipoic acid is a potent antioxidant and has the potential to prevent diabetes, influence glucose control and prevent diabetic complications such as neuropathy, nephropathy, and cataracts. In addition to the above, studies have shown that ALA may be helpful with cognitive function, heavy metal toxicity, glaucoma and liver disease.

DOSAGE: *100–200 mg three times daily*

***All the above nutrients along with Nopal Cactus, Bilberry and Holy Basil can be found in the product *GlucoSense*®, an excellent product for balancing healthy blood sugars, preventing insulin resistance and diabetes and its associated complications.

DOSAGE: *1–2 capsules three times daily with food*

## Flaxseed Oil and/or Pure Fish Oil

Essential fatty acids in the form of flaxseed or uncontaminated fish oil support healthy cell membranes by keeping them flexible with more insulin receptors thus preventing insulin resistance and improving glucose metabolism. These healthy fats also promote anti-inflammatory pathways in the body, which protect the heart, breasts and uterus. Fish oils have been shown to increase thermogenesis and decrease body fat deposition.

DOSAGE: *Take up to 2 Tbsp of flax oil daily and/or up to 4000 mg fish oil daily with a minimum of 1000 mg EPA and 600 mg DHA*

### Chaste Tree Berry - *Vitex agnus castus*
Vitex, commonly known as chastetree berry, has been traditionally used to treat menstrual irregularities to help establish a normal menstrual cycle and improve fertility. It is thought to exert hormonal activity by its action on the pituitary gland, specifically on the production of luteinizing hormone (LH). LH stimulates progesterone release after ovulation.

DOSAGE: *Take up to 400 mg daily.*
*It may take up to three months to see results.*

### Liver Support – *EstroSense®*
Supporting the liver's ability to break down hormones and fats is essential for treating PCOS, reducing excess androgens and estrogens and promoting healthy ovulation.

DOSAGE: *3 capsules twice daily*

### Adrenal Support – *AdrenaSense®*
Chronic stress increases excess androgens in the body and affects how the liver can efficiently eliminate and metabolize excess estrogens.

DOSAGE: *1 capsule three times daily*

### Vitamin B Complex + Vitamin B6
B vitamins are important for metabolizing estrogen through the liver

and vitamin B6 is specifically important for decreasing excess testosterone.

DOSAGE: *B complex – 100 mg daily, Vitamin B6 – 100 to 250 mg daily*

## Saw Palmetto – *Serenoa repens*
Saw palmetto inhibits the activity of an enzyme, 5-alpha reductase,
thereby reducing the conversion of testosterone to dihydrotestosterone,
the more potent form. This may have implications in reducing acne, excess facial and body hair, as well as hair loss from the scalp. Saw palmetto
was recently studied as part of a formula and was able to initiate a reduction in hair loss and an improvement in hair density in patients with
testosterone-related hair loss.

DOSAGE: *320 mg daily*

## CoQ10
CoQ10 is an important antioxidant and is necessary for the production
of our body's ATP, our energy fuel. CoQ10 has also been shown to have
a role in reducing fasting blood sugar. One study reported a 30% reduction in blood sugar in 31% of the patients who were given 120 mg of
CoQ10 daily for two to eighteen weeks.

DOSAGE: *100-200 mg daily*

## Calcium/Magnesium with Vitamin D
Calcium, magnesium and vitamin D are the most important nutrients
our body needs, affecting muscles, bones, thyroid, brain, heart, hormones,
colon, breast and more. Calcium and vitamin D regulation may also
contribute to the development of faulty ovarian follicle development in
women with PCOS, resulting in reproductive and menstrual dysfunction. Vitamin D plays a role in glucose metabolism and is commonly
deficient in individuals with type 2 diabetes. Supplementing with vitamin D has been shown to improve glucose tolerance, insulin secretion

and insulin sensitivity in those with diabetes. A deficiency of vitamin D may be more frequent in women with PCOS and in a small study, five of thirteen women had an overt vitamin D deficiency.

DOSAGE: *1000 mg of calcium citrate/malate, 500 mg of magnesium bisglycinate/citrate and 2000 IU of vitamin D daily*

## Probiotics - *Lactobacillus acidophilus* and *Bifidobacterium* spp.

Probiotics are known to play an important role in the maintenance of normal flora in the gastrointestinal tract. They are important in the detoxification of excess estrogens and androgens from the body through the bowel along with adequate dietary fibre.

DOSAGE: *at least 10 billion CFU daily with food*

## Licorice – *Glycerrhiza glabra*

Many women are prescribed spironolactone for excess hair growth and testosterone. Unfortunately, it does have unwanted side effects such as excess urination, weight gain, breast tenderness and dizziness.

Licorice extract has been studied for its ability to decrease the side effects associated with spironolactone.

DOSAGE: *3.5 g/day of licorice root extract standardized to 7.6% glycyrrhetinic acid*

**NOTE: Licorice extract should not be consumed by those individuals with high blood pressure.**

 **FACT – Did You Know?**

The effect of Maitake mushroom extract was explored in comparison with clomiphene citrate for its ability to induce ovulation in women with PCOS. This open trial was conducted in Japan on 80 women with PCOS. A total of 72 patients were randomized, with half receiving Maitake mushroom extract and half receiving clomiphene citrate for up to 12 weeks. The study found that the ability of Maitake extract to induce ovulation in patients with PCOS was quite impressive with a success rate of 76.9%.

## Progesterone Cream

If progesterone levels are low, a bio-identical progesterone cream may be used to offset estrogen dominance and regulate the menstrual cycle.

DOSAGE: *¼–½ tsp twice daily from Day 15 to Day 28*
***See a complementary health care professional or naturopathic doctor for specific individual dosages.*

# CONVENTIONAL MEDICINE

## Metformin

Some women with PCOS have insulin resistance. This is also found in Type 2 diabetes and results from the body not being able to use insulin properly. In many cases of Type 2 diabetes, the pancreas produces enough insulin but because of insulin resistance, sugar remains in the blood instead of being used as fuel. With the discovery of insulin resistance in PCOS, a potential treatment option with anti-diabetic drugs, such as Metformin, was explored. Metformin increases the sensitivity of the cells to insulin so that less needs to be excreted by the pancreas. With the lower levels of insulin, testosterone, androstenedione, and LH levels will decrease as well and ovulation is enhanced.

## Oral Contraceptives

The birth control pill helps to regulate irregular cycles in women with PCOS as well as assist with excess hair growth. However, the long term side effects include higher insulin levels, various nutrient depletions such as folic acid and B vitamins, as well as an increase in the risk of heart disease and breast cancer.

## Oral Contraceptives plus spironolactone

Spironolactone is a drug that inhibits the binding of testosterone to its receptors and thus decreases abnormal hair growth. Unfortunately, side effects include excess urination, weight gain, breast tenderness, fatigue and dizziness.

## Clomid – Ovulation induction

Clomid is a drug used to induce ovulation in women who want to become pregnant. Ovulation is achieved in 75 to 80% of patients, with pregnancy rates of up to 20% per ovulatory cycle. Side effects can include hot flashes, abdominal bloating, emotional effects, multiple pregnancy, ovarian cyst formation and thinning of the uterine lining.

More than six cycles of Clomid can increase the risk of ovarian cancer.

# CHAPTER 19

# PREGNANCY

Finding out that you are expecting a baby can generate an array of overwhelming emotions for most couples. These are exciting times and most women want to do everything they possibly can to ensure a healthy pregnancy for themselves and their child. Pregnancy is a time of major hormonal change which can cause emotional and physiological responses in the body. Therefore, optimal nutrition and good lifestyle choices are imperative to support a healthy pregnancy.

Pregnancy usually lasts about 40 weeks, counting from the first day of your last normal period. The weeks are grouped into three trimesters and understanding your pregnancy week by week can help most women feel more comfortable about what lies ahead.

## First Trimester (Week 1 – Week 12)
The first trimester is a time where the fetus is the most susceptible to changes in its environment. Exposure to toxins and nutritional deficiencies are most harmful during this period because of rapid growth and formation of organs. The first trimester is also when the "mom-to-be" may experience symptoms of morning sickness, nausea and vomiting. Approximately 80% of women will feel nauseated between the fourth and seventh weeks. Other symptoms may include:
- Extreme fatigue

- Tender, swollen breasts
- Cravings
- Mood swings
- Constipation
- Headache
- Heartburn
- Frequent urination.

## Second Trimester (Week 13 – Week 24)

Most women find the second trimester of pregnancy easier than the first as mom's physiology has adapted to the demands of the pregnancy. Nausea and vomiting has usually subsided but more noticeable changes are happening. The baby is growing and the abdomen expands as the baby continues to grow. As the body changes to accommodate the growing baby, some women may have:

- Body aches, especially back, abdomen, groin, or thigh pain
- Stretch marks on the abdomen, breasts, thighs or buttocks
- Darkening of the skin around the nipples
- A line on the skin running from belly button to pubic hairline
- Patches of darker skin, usually over the skin, forehead, nose or upper lip
- Itching on the abdomen, palms and soles of the feet
- Swelling of the ankles, fingers and face.

## Third Trimester (Week 25 to Week 40)

During the third trimester, final developmental milestones have been achieved such as taste buds, brain development and the maturing of kidneys and lungs. The baby gets in position, ready for labour and delivery. At this time, most women feel as if they are in the "home stretch" but the same discomforts experienced in the second trimester may continue, such as back pain. As the baby gets bigger, it puts more pressure on mom's organs as well as the spine and ligaments.

Some new changes might include:

- Shortness of breath – as the baby puts more pressure on the diaphragm and lungs
- Heartburn
- Swelling of ankles, fingers and face
- Hemorrhoids
- Tender breasts
- Belly button may protrude
- Sleep disturbances.

## FETAL RISKS

The first trimester marks a very critical time as the fetus is most vulnerable to its environment, especially toxins. The following are some examples of potential harmful chemicals in which exposure should be eliminated or minimized to protect the growing fetus.

### Alcohol

Alcohol should be eliminated before and during pregnancy since consumption may cause low birth weight, fetal alcohol syndrome, hyperactivity, poor concentration, lower IQ, heart murmurs, intellectual disability and facial abnormalities.

### Smoking and Second-Hand Smoke

When mothers smoke or expose themselves to second-hand smoke, the growing baby gets less oxygen and nutrients. This can cause low birth weights and increase the risk that the baby will have complications during the perinatal period. Cigarette smoking can expose a baby to over 4000 toxins, many of which are associated with cancer. Smoking also increases the incidence of miscarriage, sudden infant death syndrome, ectopic pregnancy and respiratory conditions such as asthma.

### Caffeine – coffee, black tea, chocolate, colas

Caffeine can cross the placenta and reach 80% of maternal blood levels in the fetus. Some studies have found that consuming caffeinated beverages (more than four cups a day) during pregnancy is associated with a shortened gestation and lowered birth weight. Caffeinated beverages should be minimized or completely eliminated to reduce the risk of miscarriage, possible birth defects and hyperactivity later in life for the child. Since caffeine is known to enter breast milk, consumption should be monitored for nursing mothers as well.

## Caffeine Content in Foods and Drinks

| | |
|---|---|
| Coffee, brewed (6oz) | 108-180 mg |
| Coffee, instant (6oz) | 60-90 mg |
| Coffee, decaffeinated (8oz) | 2-5 mg |
| Double espresso (2oz) | 45-100 mg |
| Black tea, steeped for 5 min (8oz) | 60-100 mg |
| Green tea (8oz) | 20 mg |
| Coke (12oz) | 34 mg |
| Dark Chocolate (1oz) | 40-50 mg |

### Environmental Toxins
PCBs, dioxin, phthalates, bisphenol-A, pesticides and brominated fire retardants can lead to immune deficiencies, ear infections, reproductive abnormalities, thyroid problems and estrogen-dependent conditions such as endometriosis, fibroids and breast cancer.

Solvents, cleaners, paints, nail polish remover, chemical dyes, formaldehyde and PVC should be avoided to prevent possible miscarriage.

### Heavy metals
Heavy metals such as lead, mercury, cadmium, arsenic and aluminum can lead to neurological problems, thyroid disease, learning disabilities, and risk of infertility and miscarriage.

Mercury easily crosses the placenta where it can impair the development of the central nervous system of the fetus. Avoid seafood containing high amounts of mercury such as tuna, Atlantic halibut, king mackerel, marlin, sea bass, shark, swordfish and orange roughy – Health Canada recommends that pregnant, breastfeeding and even women of child-bearing age should not eat more than 150 g of these fish *per month.* Check the Seafood Selector at www.edf.org

## Pharmaceutical drugs

Some medications such as lithium (for bipolar disorder) and tetracycline (an antibiotic) can harm the fetus. Other medications that should be avoided during pregnancy include Accutane (for acne), steroids, sulfa drugs and laxatives. It is important to discuss this with your health care professional. Most should be able to provide a full list of over-the-counter and prescription medications rated in terms of safety and side effects.

## Recreation drugs

It is important to avoid all recreational drugs before and during pregnancy. Marijuana has been linked to increased risk of miscarriages and fetal deformities. Cocaine can decrease sperm count and motility.

## Radiation

X-rays and excess radiation exposure should be avoided or minimized to prevent DNA damage and possible birth defects.

## Electromagnetic fields

Excessive exposure to EMFs from microwaves, TVs, computers, cell phones and more can increase the risk of miscarriage.

## *PREVENTION and TREATMENT – Dietary and Lifestyle*

## FOOD FACTORS

Numerous physiological changes occur during pregnancy to help with the development of a healthy fetus. Therefore, optimal nutrition and lifestyle habits are important for both mom and baby to ensure a healthy pregnancy.

- Maintain a healthy weight. Average weight gain during pregnancy is 28 pounds. Mom's weight is usually most prominent in the first half of the pregnancy while the growth of the fetus is most rapid in the second half of the pregnancy.

- Include healthy protein sources (vegetable or animal) such as hormone- and antibiotic-free chicken, turkey, fish, legumes, eggs, nuts/seeds and organic soy products. Minimize hormone- and antibiotic-free red meat to one to two times per week.
- Include calcium-rich foods - organic dairy, collards, spinach, turnip greens, black eyed peas, kale, organic soybeans.
- Green leafy vegetables and coloured fruits and vegetables are packed full of antioxidants and key nutrients. Kale, broccoli, peppers, squash, berries and many others should be included in the diet.
- Include vitamin C-rich foods such as papaya, bell peppers, strawberries, broccoli, kiwi, oranges and grapefruit.
- Include iron-rich foods - red meat, dark leafy greens, dried fruits (prunes, raisins), beans, lentils and artichokes.
- Whole grains and complex carbohydrates should be included such as brown rice, quinoa, millet, buckwheat and barley.
- Processed foods and refined carbohydrates should be minimized as well as trans fat and hydrogenated fatty foods.
- Avoid seafood containing high amounts of mercury, such as tuna, Atlantic halibut, marlin, sea bass, shark and swordfish. Consuming up to 12 oz of fish per week during pregnancy appears to be safe. However, choose fish that generally have low levels of contaminants - salmon, trout, herring, sole and char.
- Drink at least one litre of filtered water daily and mineral rich teas such as nettle, oat grass, raspberry leaf and alfalfa.

## LIFESTYLE TIPS

- Try to eat organic as much as possible. This will reduce the exposure level of pesticides for you and your baby. Check out the "Dirty Dozen" and the "Clean 15" on *www.ewg.org*
  - o HIGH in pesticides: apples, celery, strawberries, spinach
  - o LOW in pesticides: avocado, onions, asparagus, mango
- Minimize the use of plastics. Use glass instead of plastic food

containers and avoid plastic lined cans (contain bisphenol-A)

- Use glass or stainless steel beverage containers.
- Avoid non-stick cooking pans – use glass, ceramic (lead-free) or stainless steel instead.
- Use more environmentally friendly cleaning products around the house. Use low or no volatile chemicals (VOCs) paints.
- Use healthier cosmetics and personal care products – look for toxins such as parabens, phthalates and others that may be hormone disrupters.
- Get at least eight hours of sleep each night and nap during the day if necessary.
- Exercise – walk 45 minutes to an hour daily, practice prenatal yoga, stretching and deep breathing three or more times a week to prepare your body for childbirth.

## KEY SUPPLEMENTS

### Folic acid

Women who are on oral contraceptives prior to becoming pregnant may be at an increased risk of being deficient in folic acid. Low folic acid during pregnancy can lead to low birth weight, neural tube defects and possibly other birth defects.

DOSAGE: *at least 1 mg daily*

### Vitamin B12

Vitamin B12 is needed for proper homocysteine metabolism. Vitamin B12 is also important for protecting against miscarriages, neural tube defects and prevents anemia.

DOSAGE: *500 – 1000 mcg daily*

### Vitamin B3 – Niacin

Research has shown that vitamin B3 protects the nervous system and brain from free radical damage.

DOSAGE: *50 mg daily*

## Vitamin B2 – Riboflavin
Vitamin B2 is commonly deficient in pregnant women. It is involved in the activation of vitamin B6 and utilization of folic acid.

DOSAGE: *20 mg daily*

## Vitamin B1 – Thiamine
Vitamin B1 is usually low in pregnancy and healthy levels contribute to a higher infant birth weight and size. A vitamin B1 level in mom in the third trimester of pregnancy determines the amount of thiamine in breast milk later on.

DOSAGE: *30 mg daily*

## Vitamin B6
Vitamin B6 is often effective at reducing "morning sickness" – the nausea and vomiting in pregnancy that most women will experience. Women with a history of oral contraceptive use or smoking cigarettes prior to becoming pregnant have an increased risk of having low B6 status during pregnancy. Vitamin B6 may also be helpful for leg cramps and preventing toxemia of pregnancy.

DOSAGE: *100 mg daily*

## Vitamin A
Pregnant women need to be cautious about vitamin A supplementation since consuming more than 10,000 IU daily can lead to birth defects. Women who are deficient in vitamin A may be at risk of developing pre-eclampsia so it may be wise to take no more than 6,000 IU to avoid these complications. It may be best to consume higher amounts of beta-

carotene instead as it has not been associated with toxicity.

DOSAGE: *no more than 6000 IU daily*

## Vitamin C
Vitamin C is an important antioxidant and helps with the formation of collagen, a major building block of connective tissue, cartilage and bone. Vitamin C may help prevent premature rupture of membranes, prevent urinary tract infections as well as help speed up recovery and healing after a cesarean section.

DOSAGE: *1000 – 2000 mg daily or to bowel tolerance*

## Vitamin D
Vitamin D helps support healthy bones and teeth by helping to metabolize calcium. Vitamin D during pregnancy may also play a significant role in health and disease prevention. Optimal levels of vitamin D may reduce the risk of immune disorders such as multiple sclerosis, rheumatoid arthritis and chronic disease later in life.

DOSAGE: *1000 IU daily*

## Vitamin E – Mixed Tocopherols
Vitamin E is commonly deficient in pregnant women. Low levels can be associated with an increased risk of miscarriage, low birth weight, premature infants and preeclampsia.

DOSAGE: *400 IU daily*

## Iodine
Iodine deficiency during pregnancy can lead to hypothyroidism in the fetus, which can lead to developmental problems.

DOSAGE: *150 mcg daily*

## Choline
Choline is essential for brain and nerve development and improved cognitive function for the infant both early on and later in life.

DOSAGE: *150–450 mg daily*

## Chromium
Many women have low levels of chromium during pregnancy. Chromium may help prevent gestational diabetes.

DOSAGE: *100 mcg daily*

## Calcium citrate/malate
Calcium intake during pregnancy is important for increased bone density and may help prevent hypertension, leg cramps, insomnia, pain during labour and preeclampsia.

DOSAGE: *1000 mg daily*

## Magnesium bisglycinate/citrate
Supplementation during the first trimester is important for the prevention of preeclampsia, premature and low birth weight infants.

DOSAGE: *500 mg daily*

## Iron
Iron is the next most important vitamin during pregnancy after folic acid. Iron deficiency is quite common during pregnancy because the fetus draws on maternal stores. Iron supports healthy infant birth weight, size and brain development.

DOSAGE: *30 mg daily*

## Zinc

Zinc is an important vitamin for immunity and fetal growth. Zinc deficiency is associated with miscarriage, premature delivery, neural tube defects, low birth weight and toxemia of pregnancy.

DOSAGE: *20–30 mg daily*

## Bioflavonoids

Bioflavonoids are useful for women who experience recurrent miscarriages.

DOSAGE: *200 mg daily*

## Coenzyme Q10

CoQ10 is an important antioxidant for supporting healthy immune function, preventing miscarriages and improving fertility.

DOSAGE: *100 mg daily*

*\*Note: Many of the above vitamins and minerals can be found in a good quality prenatal multivitamin.*

## Flaxseed Oil and/or Pure Fish Oil

Essential fatty acids in the form of flaxseed oil or uncontaminated fish oil are important for pregnancy because they help support brain and nervous system development. Docosahexaenoic acid (DHA) and eicosapentaenoic acid (EPA) are especially important for the developing fetus – the central nervous system, brain, eyes and the immune system are all associated with an adequate intake of these essential fatty acid components during pregnancy.

DOSAGE: *Take up to two Tbsp of flax oil daily and/or up to 3000 mg fish oil daily with a minimum of 1000 mg EPA and 600 mg DHA.*

Probiotics - *Lactobacillus acidophilus* and *Bifidobacterium* spp.
Probiotics are known to play an important role in the maintenance of normal flora in the gastrointestinal and urinary tract. Probiotics also support optimal immune function as 70% of our immune cells do reside in our gut! During a vaginal birth, these bacteria populate the infant's intestines with good flora thus ensuring that the infant develops a strong immune system.

DOSAGE: *at least 10 billion CFU daily with food*

## MORNING SICKNESS
Morning sickness commonly affects 80% of pregnant women and is usually most common during the first trimester. In most cases, symptoms resolve around the end of the first trimester and do not adversely affect the health of the mother or fetus. Some women may experience a severe form of nausea and vomiting called hyperemesis gravidarum which can lead to nutritional deficiencies, weight loss, dehydration and electrolyte imbalances. These women often need to be hospitalized to replace fluids. Some women may experience nausea and/or vomiting throughout their pregnancy.

## CAUSES
Morning sickness may be linked to an increase in thyroid hormone (T4) on smooth muscle relaxation of the stomach, low blood sugar levels or nutrient deficiencies such as vitamin B6.

### *PREVENTION and TREATMENT – Dietary and Lifestyle*

### FOOD FACTORS and LIFESTYLE TIPS
To avoid symptoms of nausea and vomiting during pregnancy some common dietary recommendations include:

- Eat frequent (every two to three hours) small meals during the day
- Avoid spicy or fatty/greasy foods

- Include plenty of protein such as almonds, bean dips and nut butters for snacking in between main meals; this will help stabilize blood sugars
- Have a snack before bed (nut butter and rice crackers/cake)
- Chew on dry crackers to relieve nausea
- Drink ginger tea. (Add fresh slices of ginger root to boiling water and simmer for 15 minutes. Add honey to taste.)
- Other beneficial teas include anise, fennel, peppermint, spearmint, raspberry leaf and chamomile
- Use acupressure points. Pericardium 6 (PC6) is located three finger widths above the wrist crease on the under side of the arm between the two tendons. This relieves nausea when stimulated by massaging with your thumb, sea bands, small magnets or acupuncture treatments.

## KEY SUPPLEMENTS

### Vitamin B6
Many studies have found that pregnant women who experience nausea and vomiting have deficiencies in B vitamins, especially vitamin B6.

DOSAGE: *25-100 mg in divided doses daily*

### Ginger root – *Zingiber officinale*
Ginger root has anti-nausea and anti-vomiting properties and has been used to treat motion sickness, nausea induced by medications and morning sickness. Ginger has been reported to be as effective as vitamin B6 in clinical trials.

DOSAGE: *250 mg of ginger root powder four times daily*

## MUSCLE CRAMPING
Leg cramps are painful involuntary muscle contractions that can affect the calf, foot or both. Approximately 50% of pregnant women experi-

ence leg cramps, often striking at night during the third trimester.

## CAUSES
Possible causes of leg cramps include: lactic acid buildup, a deficiency of calcium/magnesium, poor circulation, low sodium or a vitamin B6 deficiency.

## *PREVENTION and TREATMENT – Dietary and Lifestyle*

## FOOD FACTORS and LIFESTYLE TIPS
- Increase water intake to help with excess lactic acid. Drink at least one to two litres of filtered water daily.
- Exercise daily – walking, swimming, yoga, or stretching.
- Do dry skin brushing daily to improve circulation (see **Appendix** *Dry Skin Brushing*).
- Apply heat to the affected area to relieve cramping.
- Eat potassium-rich foods such as bananas, apricots, avocado, squash, legumes and sweet potatoes.
- Seek massage therapy treatments to improve circulation.

## KEY SUPPLEMENTS

### Calcium citrate/malate
Research reports have shown the benefit of calcium supplementation for muscle cramping.

DOSAGE: *1000 mg daily*

### Magnesium bisglycinate/citrate
In a double-blind study, 73 women were randomly assigned to receive 365 mg of magnesium or placebo for three weeks. Compared to placebo, magnesium supplementation significantly reduced the severity of leg cramps.

DOSAGE: *200–500 mg daily*

## Vitamin B6
DOSAGE: *50–100 mg daily*

## Vitamin E
DOSAGE: *400 IU daily*

## Vitamin C
DOSAGE: *500–1000 mg daily or to bowel tolerance*

## VARICOSE VEINS and HEMORRHOIDS

Varicose veins and hemorrhoids can develop for some pregnant women due to softening of the muscular walls of the veins caused by hormonal changes (increased progesterone) and extra pressure on the venous system from an increase in blood volume and weight from the growing fetus.

### *PREVENTION and TREATMENT – Dietary and Lifestyle*

### FOOD FACTORS and LIFESTYLE TIPS

- Exercise – walking, yoga and other non-stressful exercise will improve circulation in the lower body.
- Increase dietary fibre in the form of ground flaxseeds, psyllium, oat bran, legumes, beets, apples and carrots.
- Eat foods high in vitamin C and other bioflavonoids to support the circulatory system and capillaries. These include berries, buckwheat, peppers, rose hips, oranges, nettles, grapefruit, onion, garlic and leeks.
- If you stand for long periods of time, wear support stockings. Take the weight off your legs by putting your feet up whenever possible. Prop your feet up at least twice daily for 15 minutes.
- Try to avoid crossing your legs, wearing high heels or sitting for extended periods of time.

**FACT - Did You Know?**

Witch hazel is known as an astringent herb, which helps to tighten tissues and reduce swelling. Witch hazel may be helpful for the relief of hemorrhoids and varicose veins. It is typically used in a sitz bath or topically for hemorrhoids and varicose veins.

## KEY SUPPLEMENTS

Vitamin C with Bioflavonoids

Vitamin C with bioflavonoids support healthy connective tissue and maintain elasticity in the veins and capillaries.

DOSAGE: *2000 mg of vitamin C or to bowel tolerance and and 1000 mg of bioflavonoids daily*

## HEARTBURN, GAS and CONSTIPATION

Hormonal changes (increased progesterone) in pregnancy soften the smooth muscle found in the walls of the digestive tract, which makes food move through at a slower rate causing gas and constipation. The softening of the muscular valve between the esophagus and stomach can cause heartburn because partially digested food can leak back up into the esophagus causing pain. As the uterus enlarges with the growth of the baby, the stomach is displaced upwards thus forcing food and stomach acid into the esophagus causing heartburn.

### *PREVENTION and TREATMENT – Dietary and Lifestyle*

### FOOD FACTORS and LIFESTYLE TIPS

* Avoid acid-causing foods such as coffee, tomatoes, greasy and spicy foods.
* Don't smoke! It irritates the stomach and is harmful to the baby.
* Chew food carefully and slowly and eat small frequent meals.
* Chew raw papaya (or in tablet form) to help digestion.
* Drink anise or fennel tea for digestive discomfort.

- Use slippery elm powder mixed with honey and water to sooth the esophagus and stomach.
- To prevent constipation, increase dietary fibre in the form of ground flaxseeds, psyllium, oat bran, legumes, beets, apples and carrots.
- Don't drink with your meals; it can dilute stomach acid and disturb optimal digestion.
- Don't lie down immediately after eating. Try not to eat past eight pm to allow food to digest properly before bedtime.

## GESTATIONAL DIABETES

Gestational diabetes develops during pregnancy due to insulin resistance resulting from the release of large amounts of hormones from the placenta. This leads to impaired blood sugar regulation thus an increase in blood sugar levels in the body.

### *PREVENTION and TREATMENT – Dietary and Lifestyle*

### FOOD FACTORS and LIFESTYLE TIPS

- Exercise 30 to 40 minutes at least three times per week. Walking, swimming, and yoga will lower blood sugar levels by stimulating the body to move glucose (sugar) into the cells, where it is used for energy. Exercise also increases the sensitivity of the cells to insulin. The result is that the body then produces less insulin to transport sugar.
- Avoid white foods (white flour, white bread, white rice and baked goods such as cookies, donuts and muffins). These foods convert too quickly to sugar in the body and increase blood glucose levels.
- Start your day off with a low GI (glycemic index) breakfast. Enjoy oatmeal with blueberries, protein smoothie or a hard-boiled egg and whole-wheat toast. Skipping breakfast sets your blood sugar on a roller coaster ride that you won't recover from all day.
- Abstain from coffee. Research confirms that caffeine appears to worsen glucose tolerance and impairs insulin sensitivity. Enjoy naturally caffeine-free herbal teas instead.

- Eat regular and frequent meals. Ensure that you have healthy protein with all your main meals to prevent blood sugar spikes.
- Avoid high glycemic foods and refined, simple carbohydrates. Include complex carbohydrates in the form of whole grains, legumes, fruits and vegetables, quinoa, brown rice and oats.

## KEY SUPPLEMENTS

### Chromium

Chromium helps potentiate the action of insulin by assisting the binding of insulin to its receptor. Chromium deficiency often results in impaired glucose tolerance and chromium supplementation seems to be helpful for those with type II diabetes and gestational diabetes.

DOSAGE: *100–400 mcg daily*

## PREECLAMPSIA

Preeclampsia, also known as toxemia of pregnancy, is a serious and dangerous condition that may develop in the third trimester. It occurs in about 5% of pregnant women developing at some point after the 20th week (five months). Symptoms include: hypertension (high blood pressure), edema/swelling, protein in the urine, severe headaches, sudden weight gain, dizziness, and changes in vision.

Preeclampsia can develop into eclampsia if not managed or treated immediately. Eclampsia can cause liver damage, breakdown of red blood cells, low platelets, convulsions and even the death of the mother and/or baby. Women with preeclampsia should be monitored every few days and if the condition worsens, often a caesarean section is performed. Blood pressure may remain high for six to eight weeks after delivery but then returns to normal.

## CAUSES

The exact cause of preeclampsia is not known but some of the following factors may play a role:

- Insulin resistance
- Being overweight
- Lack of exercise
- Excess sugar, processed and high-glycemic foods
- Increased homocysteine levels (low folic acid, B12 and B6)
- Poor blood flow to the uterus, placenta and all organs
- Nutritional deficiencies: calcium, magnesium, omega-3 fatty acids, protein
- Stress!
- Increase in free radicals and low antioxidants (low vitamin C, E, selenium, lycopene, beta carotene).

## RISK FACTORS
- Previous history or family history of preeclampsia
- Being overweight (BMI >32.3)
- Being older than 35 years of age and younger than 20
- Being pregnant with twins, triplets or other multiples
- Diabetes or strong family history of diabetes
- High blood pressure before or during pregnancy
- Low vitamin D
- First pregnancy

### *PREVENTION and TREATMENT – Dietary and Lifestyle*

## FOOD FACTORS and LIFESTYLE TIPS
- Avoid sugar, baked goods, colas and high-glycemic foods.
- Eat good fats from fish, avocado, nuts and seeds, while avoiding trans fats and hydrogenated fats from processed and fried foods.
- Eat at least 60 grams of protein daily from hormone and antibiotic-free chicken, turkey, fish, eggs, organic tofu, legumes, nuts and seeds.
- Include complex carbohydrates from fruits and vegetables, legumes, and whole grains.
- Eat foods high in magnesium – organic soybeans, tofu, buckwheat, figs, black-eyed peas, almonds, Swiss chard, brown rice, kidney

beans, Brazil nuts, beet greens, and avocado.

- Drink at least two litres of filtered water daily.
- Use a small amount of sea salt daily.
- Maintain a low-stress environment by practicing deep breathing techniques, meditation and yoga. Rest when necessary.
- Exercise 30-45 minutes at least three times per week to improve blood sugar levels and lower insulin.

## KEY SUPPLEMENTS

### Calcium/Magnesium
Calcium and magnesium help to decrease blood pressure by supporting the cardiovascular system and relaxing the blood vessels.

DOSAGE: *1000 mg of calcium citrate or malate and 500 mg of magnesium bisglycinate or citrate*

### Folic acid, Vitamin B12 and B6
All of the above three vitamins are essential for reducing homocysteine levels. High levels of homocysteine have been linked to cardiovascular disease and inflammation.

DOSAGE: *2 mg of folic acid, 1000 mcg of vitamin B12 and 100 mg of vitamin B6*

### Vitamin C and E
These two antioxidants help reduce free radicals and improve immune function thus reducing the risk of preeclampsia.
DOSAGE: *1000 mg of vitamin D and 400 IU of vitamin E as mixed toco-pherols*

### Selenium
One hundred pregnant women living in China who had risk factors of pregnancy-induced hypertension, were randomly assigned to receive 100 mcg daily of selenium or placebo for six to eight weeks. Pregnancy-

induced hypertension, gestational edema and protein in the urine were significantly lower in the selenium group.

DOSAGE: *100–200 mcg daily*

## CoQ10
CoQ10 levels have been found to be lower in women with preeclampsia than in women with healthy pregnancies.

DOSAGE: *100–200 mg daily*

## L-Arginine
Arginine is the precursor to nitric oxide, which is a vasodilator. Lower levels of nitric oxide have been found in the placenta of women with preeclampsia.

DOSAGE: *1000 mg three times daily*

## Zinc
Studies have found lower levels of zinc in women with preeclampsia than in women with normal pregnancies.

DOSAGE: *20 mg daily*

---------- CHAPTER 20 ----------

# UTERINE FIBROIDS

Uterine fibroids are slow-growing, non-cancerous growths of the uterus that occur in 20-25% of women by age 40. More than 50% of women will develop them. Also known as leiomyomas or myomas, fibroids are the most common tumour of the female reproductive tract, often leading to surgery. Uterine fibroids are composed of connective tissue and muscle that develops on the inside or outside walls of the uterus. They can feel round and firm, or be soft or rock hard, are often found in groups and can vary in size from microscopic to the size of a grapefruit. Most women are actually unaware of fibroids because they often cause no symptoms. Medical professionals may find them incidentally during a pelvic exam or prenatal ultrasound.

## SIGNS and SYMPTOMS

For those women who do experience symptoms, the most common symptoms of uterine fibroids include:

- Increased menstrual symptoms – pain, heavy bleeding, irregular periods, mid-cycle bleeding
- Anemia due to increased blood loss
- Enlarged abdomen or abdominal bloating, pressure or heaviness
- Back pain

- Excessive vaginal discharge
- Frequent urination or irritation to the bladder
- Constipation
- Pain or bleeding with intercourse
- Occasionally infertility
- Obstruction to the bowel.

The location of the uterine fibroid will influence signs and symptoms:

*Submucosal fibroids* – Fibroids that grow into the inner cavity of the uterus (submucosal fibroids) are thought to be primarily responsible for prolonged, heavy menstrual bleeding and are a problem for women attempting pregnancy.

*Subserosal fibroids* – Fibroids that project to the outside of the uterus (subserosal fibroids) can sometimes press on the bladder, causing urinary symptoms. If fibroids bulge from the back of the uterus, they occasionally can press either on the rectum, causing constipation, or on the spinal nerves, causing backache.

## CAUSES

The growth of fibroids is thought to be stimulated by estrogen. Fibroids often arise in the reproductive years and regress post-menopausally implicating estrogen as one of the main factors in the cause and growth of uterine fibroids. Peri-menopause will typically cause a growth spurt in some fibroids due to a lack in ovulation, i.e. low progesterone and excess estrogen. Research has shown that fibroids have a significantly higher concentration of estrogen receptors than normal uterine muscle. There may also be an altered estrogen metabolism within the fibroid itself leading to excess estrogen in the fibroid tissue.

Some other causes may include:

- Dietary factors

- Bowel and liver toxicity
- Hypothyroidism
- Melatonin deficiency – may predispose a woman to increased fibroid growth, as melatonin decreases numbers of estrogen receptors.
- Progesterone deficiency
- Oral contraceptive use and hormone replacement therapy
- IGF-1, a growth hormone produced in the liver, is found in higher amounts in uterine fibroid cells than in healthy uterine tissue and works in favour of estrogen to stimulate fibroid growth.
- Low physical activity and obesity.

## TESTING AND DIAGNOSIS

Uterine fibroids are often found during a routine pelvic exam. Some other common tests to assist in diagnosis include:

- Ultrasound may be used to confirm a diagnosis.
- The ultrasound will confirm size and detect the contours of the uterus. It will determine if the ureters are compressed causing enlargement of the kidneys or if the fibroid is affecting the bowels in any way.
- After the initial diagnosis, a follow-up pelvic exam or ultrasound should be carried out every four to six months to determine the rate of growth of the fibroid.

### *PREVENTION and TREATMENT – Dietary and Lifestyle*

## FOOD FACTORS

A healthy diet is vitally important when addressing any health concern. Shrinking fibroids is a challenging task and most complementary health care practitioners recognize that adopting a healthy lifestyle definitely contributes to a more positive outcome. Poor nutrition can also affect the body's metabolism and detoxification of estrogens through the liver and the bowels. Alcohol in particular, will slow down the metabolism of estrogens in the liver.

Healthy liver detoxification is essential to prevention, shrinking and halting the growth of uterine fibroids. The liver plays a critical role in the metabolism of estrogens. It converts the estradiol to estrone to estriol, a weaker form of estrogen that has very little ability to stimulate the cells of the uterus.

Saturated fats, sugar, caffeine, alcohol and junk/processed foods will interfere with the body's ability to metabolize estradiol to estrone to the weaker form estriol. Some of these foods are deficient in B vitamins or will interfere with their metabolism. This makes these important vitamins less bioavailable to the body. Remember that B vitamins are essential for healthy liver function and to help regulate estrogen levels.

Whole grains such as brown rice, quinoa, oats, buckwheat, millet and rye are excellent sources of B vitamins.

High fibre foods such as whole grains in the form of flaxseeds, hemp hearts and psyllium help the body to excrete bad estrogen metabolites through the bowel. Add 2 tbsp of ground flaxseed daily to a smoothie, on top of a salad or mix in oatmeal. *The New English Journal of Medicine* first reported the role of fibre and whole grains helping reduce estrogen levels in 1982. This study found that vegetarian women who ate a high fibre, low fat diet had lower blood estrogen levels than omnivorous women with low fibre diets.

Reduction in dietary fat intake results in a reduction in serum estradiol levels, which could influence the rate of uterine fibroid growth. The data on dietary fat and estradiol levels come from a meta-analysis published in the Journal of the National Cancer Institute. Researchers reviewed 13 studies published between 1987 and 1997 that investigated the effect of dietary fat intervention on serum estradiol levels. For both pre and post-menopausal women, the analysis revealed significant decreases in serum estradiol among women who restricted fat intake. Estradiol levels were reduced by 7.4% among pre-menopausal women and 23% among post-menopausal women. In 11 of the studies, dietary fat intake was reduced by 18 to 25%.

Increasing foods and spices that have an anti-inflammatory effect (bioflavonoid-rich citrus fruits and berries, garlic and curcumin), will help to decrease any heavy bleeding associated with fibroids.

## LIFESTYLE TIPS

- Test for and detoxify heavy metals. Heavy metals such as lead, mercury and aluminum can increase a toxic burden on the liver. This impedes healthy liver detoxification and metabolism of "bad" estrogens.
- Schedule a gentle liver cleanse at least once a year.
- Apply castor oil packs over the uterus, entire abdomen and liver two to five times per week. The castor oil pack helps move a sluggish liver, improving detoxification. Do not apply castor oil packs during menstruation or if pregnant. (see **Appendix** – *Castor Oil Pack*).
- Restore normal bowel flora by taking a probiotic.
- Ensure at least two bowel movements daily. Add flaxseeds, psyllium powder and oat bran daily to decrease circulating estrogen levels. Eat 45 grams of fibre daily (see **Appendix** - *Fibre Content of Foods*).
- Eliminate plastic containers, pesticides, PVC, cosmetics containing phthalates and parabens and toxic metals from your environment.
- Minimize exposure to the birth control pill or hormone replacement therapy.
- Manage stress!

## KEY SUPPLEMENTS

### Liver Support – *EstroSense*®

Healthy liver function is absolutely critical for the treatment of uterine fibroids and other estrogen-dependent conditions. The liver is responsible for processing the foods we eat every day but also detoxifies harmful substances from our normal metabolism and our environmental exposure. In addition, one of its most critical roles is to metabolize and deactivate hormones and its by-products. The following herbs and nutrients will support healthy hormone metabolism (specifically estrogen) through the liver thus preventing estrogen-dependent conditions:

- Calcium-d-glucarate
- Indole-3-carbinol
- Sulforaphane

- DIM
- Milk thistle
- Tumeric
- Lycopene
- Green tea extract
- Rosemary extract.

DOSAGE: *3 capsules twice daily*

## B Vitamins – Vitamin B6
B vitamins, specifically vitamin B6 are essential for proper liver function, manufacturing a number of neurotransmitters, supporting the adrenal glands and the stress response and more.

DOSAGE: *50–100 mg of a vitamin B complex ensuring at least 100 mg of vitamin B6.*

## N-acetylcysteine – NAC
NAC is a precursor or glutathione (GSH), an important antioxidant produced in the liver. NAC serves as a detoxification promoter helping with the metabolism and elimination of toxic substances from the body, including harmful estrogens and their by-products. It has very strong liver-protectant properties.

DOSAGE: *500 mg three times daily*

## Lipotropic Factors
Lipotropic factors such as inositol and choline help promote the removal of fat from the liver. They are important for optimal liver function and the detoxification of the body's wastes, metabolizing and excreting excess estrogens.

DOSAGE: *250 mg twice daily of choline and 150 mg twice daily of inositol*

## Pancreatic Enzymes
Pancreatic enzymes in the form of lipases, amylases, and proteases are usually taken with meals to relieve enzyme insufficiency symptoms such as bloating, gas, indigestion, malabsorption and nutrient deficiencies. A theory has been proposed that when enzymes are taken in between meals, they may have the ability to digest protein cell membranes surrounding abnormal growth and/or cells.

DOSAGE: *2–4 capsules taken in between meals*

## Pure Fish Oil- Omega-3 Fatty Acids
Essential fatty acids, in the form of uncontaminated pure fish oil, block the formation of PGE2 which is a messenger molecule that promotes inflammatory pathways in the body.

DOSAGE: *3000 mg fish oil daily with a minimum of 1000 mg EPA and 600 mg DHA.*

## Chaste Tree Berry - *Vitex agnus castus*
Chaste Tree Berry (Vitex) is one of the single most important herbs for supporting hormonal imbalance in women. The effect of chaste tree is on the hypothalamus/hypophysis axis in which it increases luteinizing hormone and has an effect which favors progesterone. This action prevents excess estrogen from accumulating and possibly leading to the growth of uterine fibroids.

DOSAGE: *Take up to 400 mg daily.*
*It may take up to three months to see results.*

## Probiotics - *Lactobacillus acidophilus* and *Bifidobacterium* spp
Probiotics are known to have an important role in the maintenance of normal flora in the gastrointestinal tract. They also help with the detoxification and binding of harmful estrogens in the digestive tract and eliminate them from the body through the colon.

DOSAGE: *at least 10 billion CFU daily with food.*

## Adrenal Support – *AdrenaSense*®

Assess adrenal function and restore if deficient. Adrenal fatigue can affect the balance of hormones by putting more stress on the body, especially the liver.

DOSAGE: *1–3 capsules daily*

## Thyroid Support – *ThyroSense*®

Assess thyroid health. Many women who have uterine fibroids also have low thyroid disease, which results in more available estrogen to promote abnormal uterine growth and less thyroid hormones to support healthy metabolic processes in the body.

DOSAGE: *2 capsules twice daily*

## Natural Bio-Identical Progesterone Cream

Women who are deficient in progesterone often have estrogen excess. Natural progesterone may be helpful in reducing the growth of uterine fibroids and other estrogen dominance conditions.

DOSAGE: *Take ¼ to ½ tsp twice daily from Day 10 to Day 26. Do not use during menses. Apply to inner arms, thighs or chest.*

## CONVENTIONAL TREATMENT

There are many treatments options for uterine fibroids, some of which include:

## Watchful waiting

Many women with uterine fibroids experience no signs or symptoms. If this is your case, "watchful waiting" could be the best option, applying some of the natural treatment options above. Fibroids are not cancerous and rarely interfere with pregnancy. They usually grow slowly - or not at all - and sometimes shrink after menopause when levels of reproductive hormones drop.

## Medications

Medications for uterine fibroids target hormones that regulate your menstrual cycle, treating symptoms such as heavy menstrual bleeding and pelvic pressure. Medications may include:

- *Gonadotropin-releasing hormone (GnRH) agonists.* Medications called GnRH agonists (Lupron, Synarel, others) treat fibroids by causing your natural estrogen and progesterone levels to decrease, putting you into a temporary postmenopausal state. Many women have significant hot flashes while using GnRH agonists.
- *Progestin-releasing intrauterine device (IUD) – Mirena.* A progestin-releasing IUD can relieve heavy bleeding and pain caused by fibroids. It provides symptom relief only and doesn't shrink fibroids or make them disappear.
- *Other medications.* Oral contraceptives or progestins (synthetic progesterone) can help control menstrual bleeding but they don't reduce fibroid size. Non-steroidal anti-inflammatory drugs (NSAIDs), which are not hormonal medications, may be effective in relieving the pain related to fibroids but they don't reduce bleeding caused by fibroids.

## Surgery

Surgical options are usually reserved for women who have rapidly growing fibroids, heavy and prolonged menstrual bleeding, persistent abdominal pressure/pain or urinary or bowel issues. Some may include:

- *Hysterectomy.* This operation involves the removal of the uterus and remains the only proven permanent solution for uterine fibroids from a conventional approach. A hysterectomy is major surgery since a woman can no longer have children. When a complete hysterectomy is performed, the ovaries are removed along with the uterus. Since this will bring on menopause, most women elect to keep their ovaries. If the ovaries are removed, there is the option of hormone replacement therapy.

- *Myomectomy.* In this surgical procedure, the surgeon removes only the fibroids, leaving the uterus in place. With myomectomy, there is a possible risk of fibroid recurrence.

# CHAPTER 21

# VAGINITIS

Vaginitis is an inflammation of the vagina that can result in discharge, redness, itching and pain. Vaginitis is responsible for approximately 10% of all visits by women to their health care practitioners. A recent study reported that 72% of young sexually active females had one or more forms of vaginitis. Approximately 90% of vaginitis in reproductive-age women is due to one of three organisms: *Trichomonas vaginalis, Candida albicans, or Gardnerella vaginalis.*

This chapter will be discussing the most common types of vaginitis. Less frequent causes of vaginitis include: *Neisseiria gonorrhea, Herpes simplex* and *Chlamydia trachomatis.* The vagina can also be irritated by chemicals, spermicides, allergies to condoms or to your partner's semen, hot tubs, laundry soap, topical medications, douches, perfumes, tampons and scented menstrual pads. Post-menopausal women often experience vaginal dryness and irritation caused by decreased production of estrogen (see **Menopause** Chapter).

## TYPES

### *Bacterial Vaginosis*
Bacterial Vaginosis (BV) is the most common vaginal infection and affects approximately 40 to 50% of all cases in women of childbearing

age. The organism most frequently responsible for BV is *Gardnerella vaginalis.*

Signs and symptoms of BV may include:

- Vaginal discharge that's thin and grayish white
- Foul-smelling "fishy" vaginal odour, especially after sexual intercourse
- Vaginal itching or irritation
- Pain during intercourse
- Burning during urination
- Light vaginal bleeding.

Often women have bacterial vaginosis yet show no signs of the infection and don't experience any symptoms.

### Risk Factors
Bacterial vaginosis results from an overgrowth of one of several organisms normally present in the vagina. Usually, "good" bacteria flourish and outnumber "bad" bacteria in the vagina. But when the balance of these organisms is disturbed by drugs namely antibiotics, the birth control pill and hormone replacement therapy, the "bad" bacteria overtake the "good" leading to symptoms of vaginitis.

Some other risk factors for BV may include:

- Multiple sex partners or a new sex partner
- Douching
- IUD use
- Spermicidal use
- Pregnancy
- Smoking
- Diabetes
- Lowered immunity.

### *Diagnosis*

Bacterial vaginosis is typically diagnosed through a pelvic exam of which three of the following diagnostic criteria must be present:

- A thin, frothy, gray, odorous discharge
- Vaginal pH greater than 4.5
- A wet-mount lab sample that reveals "clue cells"
- A positive "whiff" test (a fish odour detected when 10 percent potassium hydroxide is added to the discharge)

### FACT - Did You Know?

In pregnant women, BV can cause premature rupture of membranes and premature labor and is responsible for 70 to 80% of all perinatal deaths.

### *Candida Vaginitis*

The frequency of vaginal yeast infections has definitely increased in the past 20 years. According to the Centers for Disease Control and Prevention, an estimated three out of four women will have a yeast infection at some time during their lives. The increased use of antibiotics seems to be a major contributing factor for the higher incidence of candida in women. This connection between antibiotic use and yeast infections is familiar to most women. Yeast infections occur when the normal environment of the vagina undergoes a change that triggers an overgrowth of a fungal organism – usually *Candida albicans. C. albicans* can cause infections in other moist areas of your body, such as in your mouth (thrush), skin folds and nail beds. The fungus can also cause diaper rash in infants.

Signs and symptoms of Candida may include:

- Intense vulvar itching
- Pain with urination
- Pain with vaginal sex
- Redness and swelling

- Burning of the vagina and vulva
- Symptoms are typically worse the week before the menstrual period
- Watery to thick white or yellow odorless discharge like "cottage cheese"
- Vaginal pH 4 to 4.5 (normal).

It is important to note that some women who culture positive for candida do not have any symptoms of vaginitis. Candida may be a normal part of the vaginal flora until something triggers it into a symptomatic condition.

## *Risk Factors*

Five percent of women will experience recurrent yeast infections, defined as four or more confirmed candida episodes in one year. Recurrent candida vaginitis typically affects immunocompromised women with conditions such as:

- Aids
- Diabetes
- Cushing's disease
- Addison's disease
- Hypo- or hyperthyroidism
- Leukemia.

Other risk factors may include:

- Stress
- Excessive sugar in the diet
- Intestinal candidiasis
- Antibiotic use
- Pregnancy
- Oral contraceptives/hormone replacement therapy/contraceptive devices
- Estrogen dominance

- Chemotherapy/radiation
- Wearing tight clothing, nylon underwear and panty hose
- Food allergies/intolerances
- Use of steroid medications (corticosteroids, prednisone)
- Heavy metal toxicity (mercury fillings).

## Diagnosis

The diagnosis of candida vaginitis is based on the above signs and symptoms but definitively confirmed through a pelvic exam by testing a sample of the vaginal discharge. The sample of discharge is placed on a slide called a "wet mount" that is viewed under a microscope looking for yeast.

## Trichomonas Vaginalis

This is a common sexually transmitted infection caused by a microscopic, one-celled parasite called *Trichomonas vaginalis*. The organism spreads during sexual intercourse with someone who already has the infection.

Signs and symptoms of *Trichomonas vaginalis* include:

- Vulvar itching or burning pain with intercourse
- Painful urination
- Lower abdominal pain
- Vaginal redness
- "Strawberry cervix", upon examination where the cervix has a punctate and papilliform appearance. It is named because of the superficial appearance to a strawberry.
- Excess discharge that is thin, runny, yellow green or grey with a rancid odour (discharge is present in 50 to 75% of women)
- Discharge is frothy 25% of the time
- Vaginal pH 6 to 6.5.

## Risk Factors

Risk factors for *Trichomonas vaginalis* include:

- Multiple sexual partners
- Gonorrhea infections simultaneous with non-barrier birth control
- Elevated vaginal pH.

The sexual transmission rates are higher from man to woman than from woman to man.

### *Diagnosis*
Diagnosis of trichomonal infections is done through microscopic evaluation (wet prep) after a sample is taken during a pelvic exam.

The diagnosis is made by directly observing the motile parasite.

## PREVENTION and TREATMENT – Dietary and Lifestyle

## FOOD FACTORS
The treatment of vaginitis must be looked at holistically, meaning that the health of the whole body will affect the health of the vagina and its ability to ward off "bad" bacteria. The goal of treatment for vaginitis is to increase the systemic immune response, improve the vaginal immune system, restore proper balance in flora and pH in the vagina, help to decrease inflammation and irritation of the tissue and prevent recurrence of vaginitis. Optimal nutrition cannot be emphasized enough to ensure a healthy immune system – our body's defense system. Many women will benefit from anti-candida diets, but from my experience these diets should be monitored by a complementary health care practitioner as these diets can be fairly strict and stressful for someone trying it for the first time. Many times, women will self-diagnose systemic candida when it may be something completely different. It may be worth visiting a complementary health care practitioner to test stool, blood and vaginal secretions. The following dietary tips will help prevent and treat all forms of vaginitis:

- Maintain a diet low in sugar and refined carbohydrates. This includes minimizing high glycemic fruits (one serving of fruit daily), honey, maple syrup, fruit juices and alcohol.

- Avoid foods with a high content of yeast and mould, such as: mushrooms, baked goods, alcoholic beverages, cheeses and peanuts.
- Avoid dairy products since the lactose in milk can promote yeast overgrowth. Dairy products are a common food allergen that can put more stress on the immune system.
- Test for common food allergens and eliminate them. Common food allergens include dairy, gluten, egg, soy, peanuts and corn.
- Increase immune-enhancing foods. Include a multitude of coloured vegetables ensuring a balance of vitamins and minerals, for example: yellow (squash), orange (carrots/oranges), green (spinach/kale) and red (pomegranate/tomatoes). Aim for at least six to eight servings daily.
- Include herbs and spices such as ginger, thyme, oregano and garlic to boost your immune system.
- Ensure adequate protein and stick to a diet low in saturated fats, and processed foods.

## LIFESTYLE TIPS

- Wear loose clothing since tight clothing can predispose to candida.
- Wear cotton underwear versus synthetic and avoid wearing pantyhose.
- Wipe front to back after bowel movements.
- Avoid wearing bathing suits for too long after swimming. Lounging around in a wet bathing suit can predispose to bacterial overgrowth and vaginitis infections.
- Avoid pre-used towels or wash clothes.
- Avoid using artificially scented soaps in the bath or washing with heavily scented or chemical soaps.
- Consider different methods of birth control as oral contraceptives and IUDs can increase the incidence of vaginitis. Use condoms or the rhythm method.
- During an infection, consider using condoms and have your partner treated for infection as well so that you don't re-infect one another.

- Do not use any chemical sprays or scents outside the vagina.
- Avoid scented tampons, pads and toilet paper.
- Assess adrenal function as chronic stress can depress the immune system and therefore the body is more vulnerable to infections (see **Adrenal Fatigue** Chapter).

## KEY SUPPLEMENTS

### *Bacterial Vaginosis*

### Vitamin E

Vitamin E is a strong antioxidant and studies have indicated an association between vitamin E status and improved immune response.

According to a 2007 study in *The Journal of Nutrition*, deficiencies in vitamin E, among other vitamins may predispose women to bacterial vaginosis by reducing their immunity.

Vitamin E oil topically or in a gelatin capsule inserted vaginally can provide a soothing and healing effect for vaginal tissue during bacterial vaginosis as well as allergic vaginitis.

DOSAGE: *400 IU daily as mixed tocopherols*
*Insert a vitamin E suppository or gelatin capsule one to two times daily for seven or more days.*

### Vitamin A and Beta Carotene

Vitamin A and Beta Carotene are excellent antioxidants and important for healthy epithelial tissues in the body. Epithelial tissues line both the outside and the inside of the body - the skin, inside the mouth, the gastrointestinal tract and the vagina. Vitamin A and beta-carotene stimulate the immune system and the immune response in the epithelial tissues to help fight and prevent infections such as bacterial vaginosis.

DOSAGE: *10 000 IU of Vitamin A or 25 000 – 50 000 IU of beta-carotene daily.*

*Insert a vitamin A suppository or gelatin capsule daily for one week or alternate with the vitamin E for two weeks.*

## Vitamin C

Vitamin C is a powerful antioxidant and well known for its immune enhancing properties thus helping to prevent and treat infections of the vagina.

DOSAGE: *1000 mg one to four times daily or to bowel tolerance*

## Goldenseal and Oregon Grape Root

Both Goldenseal and Oregon grape root contain a compound called berberine that acts as a powerful antibacterial and immune enhancer.

This has been found to benefit not only the immune response in the vagina but also the urinary and respiratory tracts and the stomach.

DOSAGE: *500 mg two to three times daily*

## Probiotics – *Lactobacillus acidophilus* and *Bifidobacterium* spp.

Probiotics are known to play an important role in the maintenance of normal flora in the gastrointestinal tract. They also help support resistance to infections especially in the treatment of bacterial vaginosis, recurrent urinary tract infections, diarrhea, IBS and other conditions.

DOSAGE: *at least 10 billion CFU daily with food.*
*Insert Lactobacillius acidophilus suppositories vaginally or as a cream topically.*

## *Candida Vaginitis*

## Caprylic acid

Caprylic acid is a fatty acid present in coconut oil and has demonstrated the ability to inhibit the growth of candida.

DOSAGE: *250–500 mg one to four times daily, increasing gradually.*

## Garlic - Allicin

Garlic and garlic extracts have demonstrated anti-candida activity *in vitro*. Allicin is the active component found in garlic that inhibits the growth of candida.

DOSAGE: *1–2 capsules two to four times daily*

## Tea Tree – *Melaleuca alternifolia*

Tea tree oil has been studied for trichomoniasis, candida and other vaginal infections.

DOSAGE: *Tea tree wash consists of 8–10 drops of oil in one pint (500 ml) of water. Wash vaginal canal for 30 seconds one to three times a week for four weeks.*

## Apple Cider Vinegar

Apple cider vinegar is rich in natural enzymes that help encourage good flora in the digestive tract and prevent the presence of candida in the body.

DOSAGE: *Apple cider vinegar wash consists of 2 tsp of vinegar in one cup of water. Wash vaginal canal once daily.*

## Boric Acid

Boric acid can be a very successful treatment for vaginal candida overgrowth. Several studies confirm its success, ranging from 64 to 98% effective.

DOSAGE: *600 mg vaginal suppositories twice daily for three to seven days*

## Grapefruit Seed Extract

Many naturopathic doctors use grapefruit seed extract for its antibacter-

ial, antiviral and antifungal properties. It may be useful for the treatment
of candida and other microbial infections. The extract can be use topically, as a vaginal wash or taken orally.

## Immune-boosting Vitamins – ACES plus Zinc

Antioxidants such as vitamin A, beta-carotene, vitamin C, vitamin E,
selenium and zinc are excellent immune boosters and may help prevent
and treat microbial infections such as candida.

DOSAGE: *10 000 IU of Vitamin A or 25 000 – 50 000 IU of beta-carotene
daily, 500-1000 mg of Vitamin C, 400 IU of mixed tocopherols (Vit E),
100-200 mcg of selenium and 30 mg of zinc.*

## Probiotics - *Lactobacillus acidophilus* and *Bifidobacterium* spp.

Probiotics are known to have an important role in the maintenance of
normal flora in the gastrointestinal tract. They also help support resistance to infections especially in the treatment of bacterial vaginosis, candida, recurrent urinary tract infections, diarrhea, IBS and other conditions.

DOSAGE: *at least 10 billion CFU daily with food.*
*Insert Lactobacillius acidophilus suppositories vaginally or as a cream topic-
ally.*

### *Trichomonas Vaginitis*

*\*Note: many of the above treatment plans apply to Trichomonas vaginitis as
well.*

## CONVENTIONAL MEDICINE

### Estriol Cream

The use of vaginal estriol cream may be a very effective treatment for
peri- and post-menopausal women who experience chronic vaginitis
and urinary tract infections. It works by supporting healthy bacterial

levels in the vagina and helps to maintain normal vaginal tissue health.

## Bacterial Vaginosis

To treat bacterial vaginosis, one of the following medications may be prescribed:

- *Metronidazole (Flagyl, Metrogel-Vaginal, others).* This medicine may be taken orally twice a day for seven days or as a topical gel inserted into the vagina for five to seven days. To avoid the potential for stomach upset, abdominal pain or nausea while using this medication, **stay away from alcohol** for the duration of the treatment.
- *Tinidazole (Tindamax).* This medication is taken orally once a day for two to five days, depending on the prescription's strength. Tinidazole has the same potential for stomach upset and nausea as oral metronidazole.
- *Clindamycin (Cleocin, Clindesse, others).* This medicine is available as a topical cream inserted into the vagina for seven days. Clindamycin cream may weaken latex condoms and that effect persists up to five days after stopping the cream.

## Candida Vaginitis

For mild to moderate symptoms and infrequent episodes of yeast infection, the following may be prescribed:

- *Short-course vaginal therapy.* A one-time application or one-to-three-day regimen of an antifungal cream, ointment, tablet or suppository effectively clears a yeast infection in most cases. The medication of choice is from the class of drugs called the azoles - butoconazole (Femstat), clotrimazole (Canesten), miconazole (Monistat) and tioconazole (Vagistat). The oil-based nature of these agents in cream and suppository form could potentially weaken latex condoms and diaphragms. Although there are few side effecs of these topical medications, some women experience a slight burning or irritation during application.

- *Single-dose oral medication.* Sometimes a one-time single oral dose of the antifungal medication called fluconazole (Diflucan) may be prescribed.

### *Trichomonas Vaginitis*

The most common treatment for trichomoniasis is to swallow one mega-dose pill of either metronidazole (Flagyl) or tinidazole (Tindamax).

# APPENDIX

## Castor Oil Pack

A castor oil pack increases blood flow and lymphatic drainage to the area being treated. These packs also promote healing to tissues and organs underneath the skin and are of great benefit to scar tissue. Castor oil can improve digestion, immune function and reduce swelling of injured joints and extremities. It is also used in cases of menstrual irregularities, uterine fibroids, ovarian cysts and any area where there is reduced circulation.

## REQUIRED ITEMS
- Castor Oil
- Piece of pure cotton flannel to cover area being treated
- Hot water bottle
- Plastic wrap

## METHOD

Drizzle the castor oil on the dry flannel so that it is wet but not dripping.

Place flannel over area to be treated (your Naturopathic Doctor will show you where that is).

Place sheet of plastic wrap over flannel (castor oil can stain linens and clothing).

Place hot water bottle on top of plastic wrap.

Leave castor oil–soaked flannel in place for 20 to 30 minutes.

While treatment is being applied, rest comfortably (read, deep breathe, meditate).

The same flannel can be re-used several times. Store it in a glass container in the refrigerator. You may need to drizzle more castor oil before each use.

*DO NOT USE ON ABDOMEN DURING PREGNANCY OR MENSTRUATION*

## Dry Skin Brushing

As the largest organ in the body, the skin plays a huge role in detoxification and elimination. Dry skin brushing helps to keep the pores in your skin open and thus encourages the elimination of toxins and other metabolic waste products. Dry skin brushing also improves the surface circulation of blood and lymph. This results in a stronger immune system and an increased ability to bring much-needed oxygen and other nutrients to the skin.

The overall benefits of dry skin brushing include, but are not limited to:

- Improved circulation and healing
- Increased cell renewal
- A stronger immune system
- Removal of dead skin cells
- Improved detoxification.

## Required Items
- A natural (not synthetic) bristle brush or loofah. It is preferable to use one with a long handle so that you can access hard-to-reach areas.

## METHOD

It is best to do your skin brushing on dry skin, before showering or bathing, so that you can then wash off any dead skin cells.

Using circular counter-clockwise strokes, begin on the soles of your feet and move up around the ankles, calves, thighs, buttocks, abdomen, breasts/chest and back. Then proceed to the palms of the hands, around the wrists and up the arms and shoulders. You should always be brushing toward the heart.

The brush should not scratch but you should feel some friction against your skin.

Wash your brush in soap and water every two weeks to remove any accumulated debris.

## Glycemic Index of Foods

### Fruit and Vegetables

| Low | Medium | High |
|---|---|---|
| Green vegetables | Yams/Sweet potatoes | Potatoes |
| Brassica family | Raw carrots | Beets |
| Tomato | Blueberries | Parsnips |
| Apple | Grapes | Dried fruit |
| Pear | Kiwi | Pineapple |
| Grapefruit | Mango | Banana |
| Peach | Orange juice | Raisins |
| Beans (lentils, black, mung, pinto, black-eyed, chickpeas) | | |

### Grains and Pasta

| Low | Medium | High |
|---|---|---|
| Pearl barley | Corn | Couscous |
| Rice bran | Brown rice | English muffin |
| Whole rye | Oatbran/Oatmeal | French baguette |
| Wheat bran | Wild rice | Bread |
| Quinoa | Pumpernickel | Millet |
| | | Crackers |
| | | Taco shells |
| | | Corn flakes cereal |
| | | Puffed rice cereal |

*From: "The Glucose Revolution" - by: J Brand-Miller PhD, T.M.S. Wolever MD,PhD, S Colagiuri MD, K Foster-Powell*

## Fibre Content of Foods

| Food | Grams of Fibre |
|---|---|
| 1 cup of kidney beans | 15 g |
| ½ cup wheat or oat bran | 10 g |
| 1 cup of lentils | 10 g |
| 2 ½ tbsp psyllium | 10 g |
| ¼ cup of ground flaxseeds | 10 g |
| ½ cup Brussels sprouts | 4 g |
| 1/3 cup of oatmeal | 3 g |
| 1 small red apple | 3 g |
| ½ cup of kale | 3 g |
| 1 cup of raspberries | 3 g |
| ½ large pear with skin | 3 g |
| ½ fresh mango | 3 g |
| ½ cup cooked brown rice | 2 g |
| 1 slice of whole wheat | 2 g |
| 3 cups of popcorn | 2 g |
| 10 almonds | 1 g |
| 1 tbsp of Peanut butter | 1 g |
| 2 tbsp of sunflower seeds | 1 g |
| 2 ½ tbsp of Cream of wheat | 1 g |
| 1 cup of Special K | 1 g |

# REFERENCES

Gaby, Alan R. *A-Z Guide to Drug-Herb-Vitamin Interactions.* 2nd Edition. New York, NY. Three Rivers Press. 2006.

Gaby, Alan R. *Nutritional Medicine.* Concord, NH. Fritz Perlberg Publishing. 2011.

Hudson, T. *Women's Encyclopedia of Natural Medicine.* Revised and Updated. New York, NY. McGraw-Hill. 2008.

Ingram, L. *The Power of Maca.* Hillsburgh, ON. ActNatural Corporation. 2010.

Kaur, S. Dharam *et al. The Complete Natural Medicine Guide to Women's Health.* Toronto, ON. Robert Rose Inc. 2005.

Kaur, S. Dharam. *The Complete Natural Medicine Guide to Breast Cancer.* Toronto, ON. Robert Rose Inc. 2003.

Marz R. *Medical Nutrition from Marz.* 2nd Edition. Portland, OR. Omni-Press. 1999.

Murray, M. and Pizzorno, J. *Encyclopedia of Natural Medicine.* Revised 2nd Edition. Rocklin, CA. Prima Publishing. 1998.

Northrup, C. *Women's Bodies, Women's Wisdom.* New York, NY. Bantam Books, 1994.

Pelton, R. *et al. Drug-Induced Nutrient Depletion Handbook* 2nd Edition. Lexi-Comp Inc. 2001.

Pitchford, P. *Healing with Whole Foods*. Berkeley, CA. North Atlantic Books. 1993.

Silverthorn, D. *Human Physiology: An Integrated Approach*. 2nd Edition. Upper Saddle River, New Jersey. Prentice-Hall Inc. 2001.

Thorne Research Inc. *Alternative Medicine Review Monographs – Volume One*. Dover, Idaho. 2002.

Weatherby, D and Ferguson, S. *Blood Chemistry and CBC Analysis*. Jacksonville, OR. Bear Mountain Publishing. 2002.

Wilson, J. L. *Adrenal Fatigue: The 21st Century Stress Syndrome*. Petaluma, CA. Smart Publications. 2001.

*www.naturalstandard.com*

<u>Adrenal Fatigue</u>

Head, K.A. and Kelly, G.S. Nutrients and Botanicals for Treatment of Stress: Adrenal Fatigue, Neurotransmitter Imbalance, Anxiety, and Restless Sleep. *Alternative Medicine Review*. Volume 14, Number 2. 2009.

Kelly, G.S. Nutritional and Botanical Interventions to Assist with the Adaptation to Stress. *Alternative Medicine Review*. Volume 4, Number 4. 1999.

Lakshmi-Chandra, M., Singh, B.B. and Dagenais, S. Scientific Basis for the Therapeutic Use of *Withania somnifera* (Ashwagandha): A Review. *Alternative Medicine Review*. Volume 5, Number 4. 2000.

<u>Birth Control</u>

Ripley, C.H. *Contraception/Gynecology* Fall 2000.

## Breast Cancer

Anderson L, Cotterchio M, Vieth R, Knight J. Vitamin D and calcium intakes and breast cancer risk in pre- and postmenopausal women. *Am J Clin Nutr.* 2010 91(6): 1699-1701.

Baines, C. *et al.* Impact of menstrual phase on false-negative mammograms in the Canadian National Breast Screening Study. *Cancer.* 1997 Aug 15;80(4):720-24.

Bhatia N, Zhao J, Wolf DM, *et al.*: Inhibition of human carcinoma cell growth and DNA synthesis by silibinin, an active constituent of milk thistle: comparison with silymarin. *Cancer Lett.* 1999 147(1-2):77-84.

Clorfene-Casten, Liane. *Breast Cancer: Poisons, Profits and Prevention.* Monroe, ME. Common Courage Press. 1996:107.

Duthie SJ, Johnson W, Dobson VL: The effect of dietary flavonoids on DNA damage (strand breaks and oxidized pyrimidines) and growth in human cells. *Mutat Res.* 1997 (1-2): 141-51.

Hirsch, K *et al.* Effect of purified allicin, the major ingredient of freshly crushed garlic, on cancer cell proliferation. *Nutr Cancer.* 2000 38(2):245-254.

*Journal of Oncology.* Infrared Imaging as a Useful Adjunct to Mammography. September 1997. Volume 6, Number 9. *www.meditherm.com/breast_thermography_studies.htm*

Lockwood K. *et al.* Apparent partial remission of breast cancer in "high risk" patients supplemented with nutritional antioxidants, essential fatty acids and coenzymeQ10. *Molex Aspects Med.* 1994 15:S231-S240.

Love, S. *Dr. Susan Love's Breast Book.* Don Mills, ON. Addison-Wesley Publishing Co. 1995:128.

Nakagawa, H., *et al.* Growth inhibitory effects of diallyl disulfide on human breast cancer cell lines. *Carcinogenesis.* 2001 Jun 22;(6): 891-897.

National Cancer Institute at the National Institutes of Health. Mammograms Fact Sheet.
*www.cancer.gov/cancertopics/factsheet/detection/mammograms*

Scambia G, De Vincenzo R, Ranelletti FO, *et al.*: Antiproliferative effect of silybin on gynaecological malignancies: synergism with cisplatin and doxorubicin. *Eur J Cancer.* 1996 32A (5):877-82.

Whitaker, Julian. Preventing breast cancer: Let's clear up the confusion on mammograms. *Alive*, April, 1999: 16-17.

Zi X, Agarwal R: Silibinin decreases prostate-specific antigen with cell growth inhibition via G1 arrest, leading to differentiation of prostate carcinoma cells: implications for prostate cancer intervention. *Proc Natl Acad Sci U S A* 1999 (13): 7490-5.

## Cervical Dysplasia

Butterworth CE Jr, Hatch KD *et al.* Oral folic acid supplementation for cervical dysplasia: a clinic intervention trial. *Am J Obstet Gynecol.* 1992 166:803-809.

Butterworth CE Jr, Hatch KD *et al.* Improvement in cervical dysplasia associated with folic acid therapy in users of oral contraceptives. *Am J Clin Nutr.* 1982 35:73-82.

Cancer Care Ontario. *Cervical Screening: A Clinical Practice Guideline.* 2005.

Canadian Cancer Society. *www.cancer.ca*

Marshall, K. Cervical Dysplasia: Early Intervention. *Alternative Medicine Review*. Volume 8, Number 2 2003.

Niwa T, Swaneck G, Bradlow HL. Alterations in estradiol metabolism in MCF-7 cells induced by treatment with indole-3-carbinol and related compounds. *Steroids.* 1994 59:523-527.

Schiff M, Becker TM, Masuk M, *et al.* Risk factors for cervical intraepithelial neoplasia in Southwestern American Indian women. *Am J Epidemiol* 2000;152:716-726.

Thomson SW, Heimburger DC *et al.* "Effect of total plasma homocysteine on cervical dysplasia risk." *Nutr Cancer.* 2000 37(2): 128-33.

VanEenwyk J, Davis FG, Bowen PE. Dietary and serum carotenoids and cervical intraepithelial neoplasia. *Int J Cancer.* 1991 48:34-38.

## Cystitis

Falagas M, Betsi G, Tokas T, Athanasiou S. Probiotics for prevention of recurrent urinary tract infections in women. *Drugs.* 2006 66(9):1253-1261.

Head, KA. Natural Approaches to Prevention and Treatment of Infections of the Lower Urinary Tract. *Alternative Medicine Review.* Volume 13, Number 3 2008.

Karefilakis C, Mazokopakis E. Efficacy of cranberry capsules in prevention of urinary tract infections in postmenopausal women. J *Altern Complement Med.* 2009 15(11):1155.

Larsson B, Jonasson A, Fianu S. Prophylactic effect of UVA-E in women with recurrent cystitis: A Preliminary Report. *Curr Ther Res.* 1993 53:441-443.

Ochoa-Brust GJ, Fernandez AR, Villanueva-Ruiz GJ, *et al*. Daily intake of 100 mg ascorbic acid as urinary tract infection prophylactic agent during pregnancy. *Acta Obstet Gynecol Scand.* 2007 86:783-787.

Ofek I, Goldhar J, *et al*. Anti-Escherichia coli adhesion activity of cranberry and blueberry juices. *NEJM.* 1991 324:1599.

Sobota A. Inhibition of bacterial adherence by cranberry juice: potential use for the treatment of urinary tract infections. *J Urology.* 1984 131:1013-1016.

## Endometriosis

Mills DS, Vernon M. *Endometriosis. A Key to Healing and Fertility Through Nutrition.* London, Thorsons. 2002.

## Fibrocystic Breast Disease

Ghent W, *et al*. Iodine replacement in fibrocystic disease of the breast. *Can J Surg.* 1993 Oct 35(5):453-60.

Lubin F, *et al*. A case-control study of caffeine and methylxanthine in benign breast disease. *JAMA.* 1985 253(16)2388-92.

Parsay S, Olfati F, Nahidi S. Therapeutic effects of vitamin E on cyclic mastalgia. *The Breast Journal.* 2009 15(5):510-514.

Pashby N et al. A clinical trial of evening primrose oil in mastalgia. *Br J Surg.* 1981 68:801-824

## Genital Herpes

Fitzherbert J. Genital herpes and zinc. *Med J Austr.* 1979 1:399.

Gaby, AR. Natural Remedies for Herpes Simplex. *Alternative Medicine*

*Review.* Volume 11, Number 2. 2006.

Griffith RS, Norins AL, Kagan C. A multicentered study of lysine therapy in *Herpes simplex* infection. *Dermatologica.* 1978 156:257-267.

Griffith RS, Walsh DE, Myrmel KH, *et al.* Success of L-lysine therapy in frequently recurrent *Herpes simplex* infection. *Treatment and prophylaxis.*

Terezhalmy G, Bottomley W, Pelleu G. The use of water-soluble bioflavonoid-ascorbic acid complex in the treatment of recurrent herpes labialis. *Oral Surg.* 1978. 45(1): 56-62.

Centers for Disease Control and Prevention. Genital Herpes – CDC Fact Sheet. *www.cdc.gov/std/herpes/STDFact-Herpes.htm*

## Heart Disease and Stroke

Anderson JW, Johnstone BM, Cook-Newell ME. Meta-analysis of the effects of soy protein intake on serum lipids. *N Engl J Med.* 1995 333:276-282.

Burr M, Fehily A, Gilbert J, *et al.* Effects of changes in fat, fish, and fibre intakes on death and myocardial reinfarction: Diet and Reinfarction Trial (DART). *Lancet.* 1989 2:757-761.

Catanzaro, J.A. and Suen, R. Clinical Laboratory Indicators of Cardiovascular Disease Risk. *Alternative Medicine Review.* Volume 1, Number 3. 1996.

Clark, C.E. *et al.* Association of a difference in systolic blood pressure between arms with vascular disease and mortality: a systematic review and meta-analysis. *The Lancet.* Early Online Publication. January 30, 2012.

Grant, W.B. Milk and Other Dietary Influences on Coronary Heart Disease. *Alternative Medicine Review.* Volume 3, Number 4. 1998.

Heart and Stroke Foundation. Women and Heart Disease and Stroke. *www.heartandstroke.com*

Kidd, P.M. Cell Membranes, Endothelia, and Atherosclerosis – The Importance of Dietary Fatty Acid Balance. *Alternative Medicine Review.* Volume 1, Number 3. 1996.

Miller, A.L. and Kelly, G.S. Homocysteine Metabolism: Nutritional Modulation and Impact on Health and Disease. *Alternative Medicine Review.* Volume 2, Number 4. 1997.

## Hypothyroidism

Kelly, G.S. Peripheral Metabolism of Thyroid Hormones: A Review. *Alternative Medicine Review.* Volume 5, Number 4. 1999.

Patrick, L. Iodine: Deficiency and Therapeutic Considerations. *Alternative Medicine Review.* Volume 13, Number2. 2008

Gaby, A.R. "Sub-laboratory" Hypothyroidism and the Empirical use of Armour Thyroid. *Alternative Medicine Review.* Volume 9, Number 2. 2004.

## Infertility

Ana C Ruiz-Luna and Stephanie Salazar. *Lepidium meyenii* (Maca) increases litter size in normal adult female mice. *Reproductive Biology and Endocrinology.* 2005.

Gaby AR. The Role of Coenzyme Q10 in Clinical Medicine: Part II. Cardiovascular Disease, Hypertension, Diabetes Mellitus, and Infertility. *Alternative Medicine Review.* Volume 1, Number 3. 1995.

Gerasimova H. Effect of *Rhodiola rosea* extract on ovarian functional activity. *Proc of Scientific Conference on Endocrinology and Gynecology.*

Sverdlovsk, Russia. 1970 Sept 15-16. Siberian Branch of the Russian Academy of Sciences. P. 46-48.

Gustavo F. Gonzales *et al.* Effect of *Lepidium meyenii* (maca) roots on spermatogenesis of male rats. *Asian J Androl.* 2001 Sep; 3: 231-233.

Mancini A, Conte G, Milardi D, *et al.* Relationship between sperm cell ubiquinone and seminal parameters in subjects with and without varicocele. *Andrologia.* 1998 30:1-4.

Zhiping H, *et al.* Treating amenorrhea in vital energy-deficient patients with *Angelica sinensis. J Trad Chin Med.* 1986 6(3): 187-90.

Zhu, D. Dong Quai. *Am J Chinese Med.* 1986 XV (3-4): 117-25.

## Interstitial Cystitis

Interstitial Cystitis Association. *www.ichelp.org*

Kelly, GS. Quercetin Monograph. *Alternative Medicine Review.* Volume 16. Number 2. 2011.

Marshall, K. Interstitial Cystitis: Understanding the Syndrome. *Alternative Medicine Review.* Volume 8, Number 4. 2002.

## Menopause

Philp, HA. Hot Flashes – A Review of the Literature on Alternative and Complementary Treatment Approaches. *Alternative Medicine Review.* Volume 8, Number 3. 2002.

Stolze H. An alternative to treat menopausal symptoms with a phytotherapeutic agent. *Med Welt.* 1985 36:871-74.

## Menstrual Abnormallities – Amenorrhea, Dysmenorrhea and Menorrhagia

Benassi L, Barletta FP, Baroncini L, *et al.* Effectiveness of magnesium pidolate in the prophylactic treatment of primary dysmenorrhea. *Clin Exp Obste Gynecol.* 1992 19:176-179.

Harel Z, Biro FM, *et al.* Supplementation with omega-3 polyunsaturated fatty acids in the management on dysmenorrhea in adolescents. *Am J Obstet Gynecol.* 1996 174:1335-1338.

Meissner HO, Kapczynski W, Mscisz A, Lutomski J. Use of Gelatinized Maca (*Lepidium peruvianum*) in Early Postmenopausal Women – a Pilot Study. *IJBS.* 2005 1 (1): 33–45.

Ozgoli G, Goli M, Moattar F. Comparison of effects of ginger, mefenamic acid, and ibuprofen on pain in women with primary dysmenorrhea. *J Altern Complement Med.* 2009 15:129-132.

## Osteoporosis

Bischoff-Ferrari HA, Willett WC, Wong JB, *et al.* Fracture prevention with vitamin D supplementation: a meta-analysis of randomized controlled trials. *JAMA.* 2005 293:2257-2264.

Feskanich D, Willett WC, Stampfer MJ, Colditz GA. Milk, dietary calcium, and bone fractures in women: a 12-year prospective study. *Am J Public Health.* 1997 87:992-997.

Holick MF, Siris ES, Binkley N, *et al.* Prevalence of vitamin D inadequacy among postmenopausal North American women receiving osteoporosis therapy. *J Clin Endocrinol Metab.* 2005 90:3215-3224.

Miller, A.L. and Kelly, G.S. Homocysteine Metabolism: Nutritional Modulation and Impact on Health and Disease. *Alternative Medicine Review. Volume* 2, Number 4. 1996.

O'Connor, D.J. Understanding Osteoporosis and Clinical Strategies to Assess, Arrest and Restore Bone Loss. *Alternative Medicine Review.* Volume 2, Number 1. 1996.

Patrick, Lyn. Comparative Absorption of Calcium Sources and Calcium Citrate Malate for the Prevention of Osteoporosis. *Alternative Medicine Review.* Volume 4, Number 2. 1998.

Weinsier RL, Krumdieck CL. Dairy foods and bone health: examination of the evidence. *Am J Clin Nutr.* 2000 72:681-689.

## PMS

Abraham G. Nutritional factors in the citiology of the premenstrual tension syndromes. *J Reprod Med.* 1983 28:446-64.

Atmaca M, Kumru S, Tezcan E. Fluoxetine versus Vitex agnus castus extract in the treatment of premenstrual dysphoric disorder. *Hum Psychopharmacol.* 2003 18:191-195.

Head, KA. Premenstrual Syndrome: Nutritional and Alternative Approaches. *Alternative Medicine Review.* Volume 2, Number 1. 1996.

Loch E, Selle H, Boblitz N. Treatment of premenstrual syndrome with a phytopharmaceutical formulation containing *Vitex agnus-castus. J Womens Health Gend Based Med.* 2000 9:315-320.

Truss CO. The role of Candida albicans in human illness. *J Orthomolec Psychiatry.* 1981 10:228-238.

## PCOS

Armanini D, Castello R. Scaroni C, *et al.* Treatment of polycystic ovary syndrome with spironolactone plus licorice. *Eur J Obstet Gynecol.* 2007 131:61-67.

Chen J, Tominaga K, Sato Y, *et al.* Maitake mushroom (*Grifola frondosa*) extract induces ovulation in patients with polycystic ovary syndrome: a possible monotherapy and a combination therapy after failure with first-line clomiphene citrate. *J Alternative and Complementary Medicine.* 2010 12(12):1295-1299

Izumi K. Effects of coenzyme Q10 on serum MDA, other serum lipids, and fasting blood sugar level of diabetics. *Jpn J Clin Exper Med.* 1980 57:1-11

Lydic M, McNurlan M, Bembo S, Mitchell L, Komaroff E, Gelato M. Chromium picolinate improves insulin sensitivity in obese subjects with polycystic ovary syndrome. *Fertil Steril* 2006 86:243-246.

Marshall, K. Polycystic Ovary Syndrome: Clinical Considerations. *Alternative Medicine Review.* Volume 6, Number 3. 2001.

Raghuramulu N, Raghunath M, Chandra S, et al. Vitamin D improves oral glucose tolerance and insulin secretion in human diabetes. *J Clin Biochem Butr.* 1992 13:45-51.

Schottner M, Gansser D, Spiteller G. Lignans from the roots of *Urtica dioica* and their metabolites bind to human sex hormone binding globulin. *Planta Med.* 1997 63(6): 529-532

Thys-Jacobs S, Donovan D, Papadopoulos A, *et al.* Vitamin D and calcium dysregulation in the polycystic ovarian syndrome. *Steroids.* 1999 64:430-435.

## Pregnancy

Dahle LO, Berg G. Hammar M, *et al.* The effect of oral magnesium substitution on pregnancy-induced leg cramps. *Am J Obstet Gynecol* 1995 173:175-180.

Dotterud C, Storro O, Johnsen R, Oien T. Probiotics in pregnant women to prevent allergic disease: a randomized, double-blind trial. *British Journal of Dermatology.* 2010 163:616-623.

Han L, Zhou SM. Selenium supplement in the prevention of pregnancy induced hypertension. *Chin Med J.* 1994 107:870-871.

Merkel RL. The use of menadione bisulfite and ascorbic acid in the treatment of nausea and vomiting of pregnancy: a preliminary report. *Am J Obstet Gynecol.* 1952 64:416-418.

Mills JL, Graubard BI, Harley EE, *et al.* Maternal alcohol consumption and birth weight. How much drinking during pregnancy is safe? *JAMA.* 1984 252 1875-1879.

Ozgoli G, Goli M, Simbar M. Effects of ginger capsules on pregnancy, nausea and vomiting. *J Alternative and Complementary Medicine.* 2009 15(3):243-246

Qvist I, Abdulla M. Jaerstad M. Svensson S. Iron, zinc and folate status during pregnancy and two months after delivery. *Acta Obste Gynecol Scand.* 1986 23:725-730.

Simpson J, Bailey L, Pietrzik K, Shane B, Holzgreve . Micronutrients and women of reproductive potential: required dietary intake and consequences of dietary deficiency or excess. Part 1-Folate, Vitamin B12, Vitamin B6. *J Matern Fetal Neonatal Med.* 2010.

Wright JT, Waterson EJ, Barrison IG, *et al.* Alcohol consumption, pregnancy and low birthweight. *Lancet.* 1983 1:663-665.

## Vaginitis

Ankri S, Mirelman D. Antimicrobial properties of allicin from garlic. *Microbes Infect.* 1999 Feb 1(2): 125-9.

Caporaso N. Smith SM, Eng RHK. Antifungal activity in human urine and serum after ingestion of garlic (Allium sativum). *Antimicrob Agents Chemother.* 1983 23 700-702.

Catanzaro JA, Green L. Microbial Ecology and Probiotics in Human Medicine Part II. *Alternative Medicine Review.* Volume 2, Number 4. 1996.

Hammer KA, Carson CF, Riley TV. *In vitro* activity of essential oils, in particular *Melaleuca alternifolia* (tea tree) oil and tea tree oil products, against *Candida* Spp. *J. Antimicrob Chemother.* 1998 Nov 42 (5): 591-95.

Hammer KA, Carson CF, Riley TV. *Melaleuca alternifolia* (tea tree) oil inhibits germ tube formation by *Candida albicans. Med Mycol.* 2000 Oct 38 (5): 355-62.

Jovanovic R, Congema E, Nguyen H. Antifungal agents vs boric acid for treating chronic mycotic vulvovaginitis. *J Rep Med.* 1991 36(8): 593-97.

Neuhauser I. Successful treatment of intestinal moniliasis with fatty acid-resin complex. *Arch Intern Med* 1954;93:53-60.

Wang Y, Reifer C, Miller L. Efficacy of vaginal probiotic capsules for recurrent bacterial vaginosis: a double-blind, randomized, placebo-controlled study. *Amer J Obst/Gyn.* 2010 120.1-120.6

# RESOURCES

## Naturopathic Colleges and Organizations

Canadian Association of Naturopathic Doctors (CAND)
20 Holly Street, Ste 200
Toronto, Ontario
M4S 3B1
(416) 496-8633
1-800-551-4381
*www.cand.ca*

Canadian College of Naturopathic Medicine
1255 Sheppard Avenue East
Toronto, Ontario
M2K 1E2
(416) 498-1255
*www.ccnm.edu*

American Association of Naturopathic Physicians
4435 Wisconsin Avenue, NW Suite 403
Washington, D.C.
20016
(202) 237-8150
1-866-538-2267
*www.naturopathic.org*

Bastyr University
14500 Juanita Drive NE
Kenmore, WA
98028-4966
(425) 823-1300
*www.bastyr.edu*

National College of Naturopathic Medicine
049 SW Porter Street
Portland, Oregon
97201
(503) 552-1555
*www.ncnm.edu*

Southwest College of Naturopathic Medicine
2140 East Broadway Rd.
Tempe, Arizona
85282
(480) 858-9100
*www.scnm.edu*

University of Bridgeport
126 Park Avenue
Bridgeport, Connecticut
06604
1-800-392-3582
*www.bridgeport.edu*

Health Action Network Society
202-5262 Rumble Street
Burnaby, BC
V5J 2B6
(604) 435-0512
*www.hans.org*

## Laboratory Testing

Hormones (blood, urine, saliva), blood tests, ELISA allergy testing, heavy metal/environmental toxicity testing, stool tests.

Rocky Mountain Analytical
Unit A 253147 Bearspaw Road NW
Calgary, Alberta
T3L 2P5
(403) 241-4513
*info@rmalab.com*

Meridian Valley Lab
801 SW 16th Street, Suite 126
Renton, Washington
98057
(425) 271-8689
1-855-405-8378
*www.meridianvalleylab.com*

Doctor's Data Inc.
3755 Illinois Avenue
St. Charles, Illinois
60174-2420
1-800-323-2784
*www.doctorsdata.com*

Genova Diagnostics
63 Zillicoa Street
Asheville, NC
28801
1-800-522-4762
(828) 253-0621
*www.gdx.net*

SpectraCell Laboratories
10401 Town Park Drive
Houston, Texas
77072

1-800-227-5227
(713) 621-3101
*www.spectracell.com*

## Breast Screening

Breast Thermography

Medical Thermography International Inc.
Suite 8-410 – 9251 Yonge Street
Richmond Hill, ON
L4C 9T3
(905) 770-7458
1-866-242-5554
*www.medthermonline.com*

Valentus Clinics
Oak Bay Professional Building
#103 – 1625 Oak Bay Avenue
Victoria, BC
V8R 1B1
(250) 590-5090
*www.valentusclinics.com*

## Recommended Reading

*www.mercola.com*

Eating Alive II
*Dr. John Matsen, ND*

The Magnesium Miracle
*Dr. Carolyn Dean, MD, ND*

Healing with Whole Foods
*Paul Pitchford*

The Wisdom of Menopause
*Dr. Christiane Northrup, MD*

Women's Bodies, Women's Wisdom
*Dr. Christiane Northrup, MD*

Mother-Daughter Wisdom
*Dr. Christiane Northrup, MD*

The Complete Natural Medicine Guide to Women's Health
*Dr. Sat Dharam Kaur, ND*

Women's Encyclopedia of Natural Medicine
*Dr. Tori Hudson, ND*

The Complete Natural Medicine Guide to Breast Cancer
Dr. Sat Dharam Kaur, ND

Encyclopedia of Natural Medicine
*Dr. Michael Murray, ND and Joseph Pizzorno, ND*

The Hormone Diet
*Dr. Natasha Turner, ND*

Fat Wars
*Brad King*

Beer Belly Blues
*Brad King*

99 Things You Wish You Knew Before Losing Fat 4 Life
*Brad King*

8 Weeks to Vibrant Health
*Dr. Hyla Cass, MD*

Vitamin K2 and the Calcium Paradox: How a Little Known Vitamin
Could Save Your Life
*Dr. Kate Rheaume-Bleue, ND*

The Bone-Building Solution
*Sam Graci*

The Clear Skin Diet
*Dr. Alan Logan, ND and Dr. Valori Treloar, MD*

The Power of Maca
*Lorrie Ingram*

Stop Being Stopped
*Dr. Karen Lee Paquette, ND*

Adrenal Fatigue: The 21st Century Stress Syndrome
*Dr. James L. Wilson, ND, DC, PhD*

The Brain Diet
*Dr. Alan Logan, ND*

Wheat Belly
*Dr. William Davis, MD*

The Thrive Diet
*Brendan Brazier*

## Great Recipes and Cookbooks

Meals that Heal Inflammation
*Julie Daniluk R.H.N.*
*www.juliedaniluk.com*

The Whole Life Nutrition Cookbook
*Alissa Segersten and Tom Malterre, MS, CN*
*www.nourishingmeals.com*

Quinoa 365: The Everyday Superfood
*Patricia Green and Carolyn Hemming*

Rebar: Modern Food Cookbook
*Audrey Alsterburg and Wanda Urbanowicz*

Thrive Foods: 200 Plant-Based Recipes for Peak Health
Brendan Brazier
*www.brendanbrazier.com*

The Detox Diet
*Dr. Elson M. Haas, MD*

Hollyhock Cooks
*Solomon Jolar*

My Father's Daughter
*Gwyneth Paltrow and Mario Batali*

Make it Fast, Cook it Slow: The Big Book of Everyday Slow Cooking
*Stephanie O'Dea*

More Make it Fast, Cook it Slow: 200 Brand-New Budget-Friendly, Slow-Cooker Recipes
*Stephanie O'Dea*

Cook4Seasons
*www.cook4seasons.com*

Gluten-free Goddess
*www.glutenfreegoddess.blogspot.com*

Simply Recipes
*www.simplyrecipes.com*

101 Cookbooks
*www.101cookbooks.com*

# NOTES